Your Type 2
Diabetes Lifeline

For Type 2 Diabetics, Pre-diabetics, and Borderline Diabetics

---

Reverse Type 2 Diabetes in One Month or Two Months—Your Choice

---

Lose Weight, Live Healthier
and Banish Type 2 Diabetes

By Rick Mystrom

PUBLICATION
CONSULTANTS
We Believe In The Power Of Authors

PO Box 221974 Anchorage, Alaska 99522-1974
books@publicationconsultants.com—www.publicationconsultants.com

Testimonials

Praise for Rick Mystrom's Books on Diabetes

"I heard you speak on diabetes and bought your book. 20 pounds gone, off diabetes meds and blood Pressure meds, no more tums. THANK YOU, and God Bless You."

Robert Maxon, Anchorage, Alaska

"This past July my morning fasting scores averaged 218 mg/dl, and I was losing ground. I began reading your book and implementing the ideas in it at the end of July and in early August. Today is August 21. My average morning fasting score so far in August has been 137, and my score has been normal on three mornings. This morning my fasting score was 88." "…I have not had a score as low as today's since at least 2008."

Ben Muse, Juneau, Alaska

"I can't say enough about how your book helped me and my husband. We turn the TV off and read it out loud together. I've lost 45 pounds and my husband has lost 15 pounds."

Laura, Colorado

"I'm not a diabetic but like many people I weighed a little more than I wanted to. I had heard so much about how people had lost weight when they followed Rick Mystrom's advice for diabetics, I decided to follow it. I lost 20 pounds in four months but most important it's easy to maintain my new, lower weight. I'm a believer."

Rick Pollock, Anchorage, AK

"I want you to know Rick that your advice saved my father's life. Thank you. Thank you. Thank you."

Denise Trutonic, Anchorage, Alaska

"Your book, *What Should I Eat,* is so well-written and understandable. It is the best book I've ever read on diabetes. As soon as I finished it I went out and bought another book for a friend. Now I keep going back to your book and I'm doing great now."

Carol Childs, Type 2 diabetic, Anchorage, Alaska

"Thanks to Rick Mystrom, I've changed my eating style and lost 34 pounds. It wasn't fast but it was steady and easy to keep off. My A1C* has gone from 10 to 7. I'm off all my medications now except for one. Thank you Mr. Mystrom."

Rabbi Greenberg, Anchorage, Alaska

"…the best explanation ever of the difference between Type 1 and Type 2 diabetes."

Kim Erickson, Willow, Alaska

---

* A1C is a measure of one's blood sugar for the previous 60-90 days. It's a reflection of how well one is managing diabetes. A lower number is better.

"I've been reading your book. I LOVE IT. I will never look at food the same way again. I've already lost 7 pounds. It was so easy to lose I fully expect I will never regain that weight and will lose more."

Kathleen Madden, Anchorage, Alaska

"I have been a Type 2 Diabetic for almost 16 years and insulin dependent for about half that time. The graphs [in Rick Mystrom's book, *What Should I Eat*] are the first of their kind I have ever seen and bring an "ah ha" moment in understanding the effect of (certain) carbohydrates on blood sugar levels. I highly recommend this book."

John Eckheard, Pomona, California

"I saw Rick on TV and his message really clicked with me. I am not diabetic but have struggled with my weight all my life. This is by far the most detailed and intelligent explanation of the ill effects of bad carbs on weight gain I have ever seen. I have followed this eating plan for 2 weeks and have already lost 9 lbs. but best of all I have the knowledge to understand why I need to eat this way for health and to avoid diabetes. Thank you Rick."

Melinda M. Hofstad

"Your book is well written, concise, and to the point, especially the graphs and illustrations to promote a healthy lifestyle. I take pride that an Alaskan has made such a contribution. I am recommending your book to my family and friends. Thank you for your contribution to my ongoing battle not to become a diabetic and to control my weight. (9)"

William M. (Bill) Bankston, Anchorage, Alaska

"Having my Dr. tell me that I might have Diabetes really woke me up. I knew I needed help. Rick Mystrom's book, *What Should I Eat* from the start was clear, to the point, and extremely informative. Who would have thought a book about a disease would be so engaging! I never skipped a page."

Robert Herndon, Roseville, California

"As parents of a recently diagnosed Type 1 Diabetes son, Rick Mystrom's book has not only profoundly impacted his diet but has changed the rest of our family's approach to food. Rick has given us a major contribution that will improve the American diet, leading to a higher quality of life for all. Thank you, Rick!"

Bill and Jean Bredar, Anchorage, Alaska

"Your Book has sprouted wings and is flying off the shelves."

Sally McCollor, Providence Hospital Gift Shop, Anchorage, Alaska

"Bravo! ...A powerful message that will help so many people—now and forever. Well done!"

Malcom Roberts, Author, Alaskan Leader

Testimonials from Medical Professionals

"I believe the overwhelming message of this book is how priceless a positive attitude is in living a great life. Rick's optimism clearly played a dramatic role in his many successes, including how well he has managed a potentially devastating disease. As an ophthalmologist, I have never seen anyone with type 1 diabetes without any evidence of eye damage after a few decades, let alone fifty years after diagnosis! Rick's story is an example for anyone, diabetic or not, to take charge of the challenges in life rather than letting them take charge of you."

Dr. Griff Steiner MD, Opthalmology

"Rick Mystrom never let diabetes prevent him from accomplishing everything he wanted in life: good health, success in business, community service, family, and politics. Rick Mystrom knew that understanding his disease was crucial to his health. He has become one of the most knowledgeable persons living with diabetes in my extensive practice and frequently serves as a role model and authoritative resource for others."

Jeanne R. Bonar, MD, FACP, FACE
Endocrinology, Internal Medicine

"It is the patient, not the doctor who manages diabetes." Rick Mystrom is the gold medal winner for controlling his Type 1 Diabetes. He has become so skilled that he can adjust his insulin level when he sees the meal he is going to eat. His results: no complications from his long history of disease. He is the expert, I am the learner."

Thomas S. Nighswander MD MPH,
Assistant Regional Clinical Dean, Alaska WWAMI Program, Anchorage, Alaska

"I've been reading books on diabetes since 1974. Your book is the best written book on diabetes I have ever found. After I read your book, I bought four more to loan out to members of my church."

R. Clinch RN BSN, Wasilla, Alaska

"If every newly diagnosed diabetic, regardless of type, could adopt Rick's two premises: having a positive attitude about living with diabetes and taking personal responsibility for modifying your food intake… The improvement in the quality of life would be outstanding."

Sue Sampson RN, BSN, Anchorage, Alaska

"You are to be commended for taking the time to document all your personal food reactions to show the downside of hi-carb foods. Your book should be a best seller!"

Pat DeVoe, RN, BSN,
Diabetes Action Research and Education Foundation, Bethesda, MD

Two Encouraging and Helpful Stories

Dear Mr. Mystrom,

It was a great pleasure to meet you in Anchorage on Wednesday, and to have the opportunity to tell you how helpful your book, *What Should I Eat* (2nd edition), has been in helping me make progress on my diabetes.

This past July my morning fasting scores averaged 218 mg/dl, and I was losing ground. I began reading your book and implementing the ideas in it at the end of July and in early August. Today is August 21. My average morning fasting score so far in August has been 137, and my score has been normal on three mornings. This morning my fasting score was 88. I have not had normal scores since July 2010, and I have not had a score as low as today's since at least 2008. I was able to make this progress in about three weeks, despite spending 10 days traveling. I am confident that I will be able to continue to make progress.

I was diagnosed with Type 2 diabetes in the summer of 2001. While I kept my fasting sugars at normal levels with diet changes for several years, I eventually lost focus and the sugars gradually rose. I have been taking 100 mg of Januvia daily now for several years. My doctor was beginning to talk about using insulin.

Your book helped me in a number of ways:

> You were very credible, based on your years of experience, the care with which you carried out the tests you had done, and the practical tone throughout.

> Because you were credible, your optimism was persuasive. After reading, I decided that I would set myself the goal of reaching normal scores, and of going off the Januvia. Based

on my experience in the last three weeks, I'm confident that I will be able to do that.

Based on my reading I decided to go from testing once a day to testing five times a day, spread throughout the day. This gives me a much better idea of the pattern of blood sugars during the day, and the feedback helps keep me conscious of the impact of my eating.

The six-food group model was a very helpful one. I used it to largely eliminate sugary and starchy carbohydrates from my diet. The need to discriminate between different fruit carbohydrates and to pay attention to the interaction of fats with starches and proteins, was new information for me and very helpful.

The idea that diet counted for 80% and activity and exercise counted for 20% (approximately) was helpful in setting priorities.

Thank you very much for your work in sharing your knowledge of diabetes. Your book will have a big impact on my life.

All the best,
Ben Muse, Juneau

Rick

I can't say enough about how much your book helped me and inspired me. In 2013 I left my job with an airline as a flight attendant when I left, my weight was under control and my health was good. Soon after I left I began eating things I didn't normally eat, including a diet high in (starchy) carbohydrates.

I soon went from a size 8–10 and about 139 lbs. to almost 190 and a size 16. More concerning than the effect it had on my self-worth was the effect it had on my health. I was told for the first time ever that my A1C was elevated and I was a pre-diabetic.

Having lived with a husband for almost 26 years who was a type 2 diabetic, had poor control, and has many health consequences as a result, that frightened me more than I can tell you.

Your son, after hearing about my husband's diabetes, sent us your book. I was so excited reading it I would ask my husband to mute the TV and I'd read the book out loud. We both committed to trying the diet in your book. To date, my husband has lost almost 15 pounds and I have lost almost 45.

We both feel better, and although we don't know for sure the results of new A1C tests yet, we feel confident the test will reflect how much better we look and feel.

Thank you for writing the book!

Sincerely,
Laura and Alan Jacques, Colorado

ISBN: 978-1-59433-719-2

eBook ISBN Number: 978-1-59433-720-8

Library of Congress Number: 2017945479

Manufactured in the United States of America.

Disclaimer

This book is intended as a reference volume only, not as a medical manual. The information contained herein is intended to help you make informed decisions about your health, weight and diabetes management. It is not intended as a substitute for any treatment prescribed by your doctor.

Mention of specific organizations or authorities, or books does not imply endorsement by their authors or publishers.

Table of Contents

Chapter 3

The Simple Science of Reversing
Type 2 Diabetes and Losing Weight

Chapter 4

The New and Better Way for Diabetics to Categorize Foods

Chapter 5

Graphics of Good Foods and Bad Foods for Type 2 Diabetics

Sweet Carbohydrates

Starchy Carbohydrates

Fruit Carbohydrates

Fruit Juices

Vegetable Carbohydrates

Protein and Fat

Good Meals, Bad Meals

Yogurt

Chapter 6

Some Tips for Eating Out

Preface

How Can a 53-Year Type 1 Diabetic Know How to Reverse or Avoid Type 2 Diabetes?

I'm a Type 1 diabetic. I was diagnosed at 20 years of age and I'm now 73. I've had Type 1 diabetes for 53 years and have no health problems. I'm very likely healthier now because of diabetes than I would have been without diabetes.

A few years ago I took a stress test that showed me equivalent to an "active 42-year-old"—26 years below my chronological age at that time. The result of that test as well as my generally excellent health are primarily the results of eating right.

What Does Eating Right Mean?

Eating right is not the way the government has told us to eat since the Food Pyramid was first introduced in 1980. That Food Pyramid was the result of the work of the Senate Select Committee on American Dietary Habits formed in 1977 and chaired by Senator George McGovern. The conclusions of that committee became the basis for the creation of the Food Pyramid. The Food Pyramid became a core part of the health and nutrition curriculum in America's elementary through postsecondary schools. Ten years after its creation it had become the unquestioned authority for healthy eating. Ten years after its creation also marked the beginning of America's obesity and Type 2 diabetes epidemic.

The government has finally—but very quietly—admitted the Food Pyramid was wrong. They have changed it to what is called "My Plate"—still wrong, but somewhat better.

I haven't learned to eat right by following the Food Pyramid or by reading what others have written about eating right. I've learned based on 60,000 blood sugar tests I've given myself after nearly every meal I've eaten and every snack I've had for the past 35 years. In this book, I share my findings with you.

Physician ... Heal Thyself

Although I'm a Type 1 diabetic, this book is for Type 2 diabetics, borderline diabetics, pre-diabetics, anyone who wants to avoid becoming diabetic, *and anyone who wants to lose weight.*

The very first question you should ask me is simply this: If I've learned how to reverse (or cure) Type 2 diabetes, why don't I cure myself?

The answer is simple. Type 1 and Type 2 diabetes are two very different versions of the same disease.

Type 1 Diabetes

Type 1 diabetes is most often diagnosed between birth and about age 25. It is not related to eating or exercise habits.

The pancreas just stops producing insulin, which is the hormone that allows the glucose from food that has been eaten to get from the bloodstream to the cells for energy. Without insulin, the glucose can't get out of the bloodstream into the cells as energy for immediate use or for storage for future use. This storage is *short term storage* in the liver or *longer-term storage* around the belly, hips, legs, arms, and butt—all the places you don't want it.

Within the constraints of today's technology, Type 1 is not curable but it is very manageable. And good management allows for a healthy, productive, and long life—as I have experienced.

Type 2 Diabetes

Type 2 diabetes is different. It is typically—but not always—diagnosed at a later age. Most commonly 40s through 70s or even 80s. It is usually associated with eating the wrong foods over a period of time combined with a relatively inactive lifestyle.

Because of less-than-healthy eating habits, the quantity of glucose (sugar)* entering the bloodstream is high and requires the pancreas to produce more insulin to get the blood sugar back to normal levels. In nonmedical terms, if the quantity of glucose entering the bloodstream is higher than normal the pancreas must work harder than normal to produce enough insulin. The pancreas is in effect overworked and eventually can't produce enough insulin to get all the excess glucose out of the bloodstream into the cells.

If blood sugars have been high for days, weeks, or months, larger amounts of insulin are required to bring the level of blood sugar down to normal, which is most often defined as 75–105 milligrams per deciliter (Mg/Dl). These large amounts of insulin required to initially bring blood sugars down to normal levels are often referred to as insulin resistance, which gives some Type 2 diabetics license to say, "Well, it's not my eating habits, I'm just insulin resistant." Please don't buy into that as an excuse for high blood sugars until you finish reading this book.

If you don't bring your blood sugars down to normal levels now, you'll have to deal later with all the serious complications brought on by continually high blood sugars. (For details of these potential complications and avoiding them, see chapter 2.)

---

* Blood sugar and blood glucose are terms that are commonly used interchangeably and are used that way in this book.

Unlike Type 1 Diabetes, *Type 2 Is Reversible*

That's what this book is about—reversing Type 2 diabetes in one or two months and avoiding all the devastating complications and early death associated with Type 2 diabetes.

Whether you call it reversing Type 2 diabetes or curing Type 2 diabetes, the effect is the same. You'll feel better, look better, and increase your lifespan—and more important, you'll increase your health span.

Desert Island Parable

Here's a story I use periodically in my speeches. By the time you finish this book you'll fully understand and appreciate the truth of this short parable.

A Type 1 diabetic and a Type 2 diabetic are marooned on a desert island. Neither has any insulin; however, they do have a way to make fires and the island does have catchable fish, edible plants, and drinkable water.

Despite access to the nourishment needed to survive, but with no insulin, the Type 1 diabetic would be dead in a month. In that same length of time, the Type 2 diabetic would be cured.

Now why, in this parable, do I say Type 2 diabetes would be reversed (cured) in one month but in the subtitle of this book I say, "Reverse Type 2 Diabetes in One or Two Months"?

AUTHOR'S NOTE:

I use the word "cure" in the parable because having normal blood sugars is the very definition of a nondiabetic. Some may argue that "cure" is the wrong word because even if blood sugars are normalized, the former diabetic may be more susceptible to becoming a Type 2 diabetic again if old habits return. But whatever it's called "cured" or "reversed" the likelihood of diabetic complications is dramatically diminished and a longer, healthier life is the result.

The answer is simply: *"Reality."* It's unrealistic to believe anyone whose eating habits have contributed to Type 2 diabetes can instantly change those habits to eating only fish and plants, and drinking only water. That *would* cure or reverse Type 2 diabetes in *one month* but you likely cannot do that and you certainly couldn't realistically sustain that type of eating over a period of years.

The good news is you don't have to make that extreme change in eating to cure or reverse your Type 2 diabetes. *All you need to do is eat more of the foods that do not raise your blood sugars significantly and less of the foods that do raise your blood sugar significantly.* Doing that will reduce the amount of insulin that your overworked pancreas must produce and allow that pancreas to produce sufficient insulin to normalize your blood sugars.

Reversing Type 2 diabetes and normalizing blood sugars can be done in one month or two months by applying what you'll learn in this book.

To reverse Type 2 diabetes in *one month* requires serious motivation and a commitment to applying—without exception—the new eating patterns you'll learn in this book.

To reverse Type 2 diabetes in *two months* is much easier and doesn't require absolute perfection in your new eating patterns. In my speeches, I often tell people, "you don't need to be perfect in your new eating patterns, you just need to be good."

How Do I Know This?

I've done something that only a Type 1 diabetic whose body produces no insulin can do—something that to my knowledge has never been done before and certainly has never been published before—and for good reason.

For three years, I conducted, recorded, and graphed self-administered blood sugar tests to give structure and specificity to the 60,000 tests I had already given myself. By doing this I visually show in chapter 5 what foods and combinations of foods contribute to high blood sugars, pancreas burden, and weight gain. Conversely, I also show what foods and combinations of foods contribute to low blood sugars, pancreas relief, and weight loss.

My Research Protocol for Developing the Graphs

I would eat the food I wanted to test and then for 90 minutes, I didn't give myself any insulin and let the food or food combinations increase my blood sugar until I gave myself an appropriate amount of insulin at 90 minutes.

To assure the most accurate results, I adhered to a consistent protocol in giving myself these tests: stable starting blood sugars, consistent starting levels, consistent times of day, and consistent situations.

Why hasn't it ever been done before? It's simply because researchers don't want to ask Type 1 diabetics to eat foods—both good and bad for diabetics— and have those subjects not take a shot of insulin for 90 minutes. It's not healthy.

I was willing to do that to myself because I believe it will help millions of people around the world live healthier, longer lives.

That's why this book is different from anything else that's ever been written about eating right, lowering blood sugar, and losing weight. This book isn't based on theories or on what other people and authors have written or conjectured, it's based on the blood tests I've given myself after eating thousands of different foods and combinations of foods over the past 35 years since self-testing has been available.

Results of the Tests

These tests have given me the information I've needed to live a healthy, happy, productive life with Type 1 diabetes for over 53 years. Now at age 73, I'm healthier than most people 20–25 years younger than I am.

These graphs also provide the core of the information Type 2 diabetics need to normalize their blood sugars, get rid of all symptoms of Type 2 diabetes—and as a bonus lose weight and live healthier. Even more, the graphs will be instrumental in helping millions of borderline diabetics and nondiabetics lose weight and avoid ever getting diabetes in the first place.

For me, blood sugar testing was my research. But as often happens in research, when you're looking for one answer, you sometimes find another. I was trying to pinpoint the impact of food and activity on my blood sugar but *what I discovered was how to reverse or cure Type 2 diabetes and how to lose weight.*

Introduction

Your Opportunity for a Longer, Healthier Life

Few—if any—diseases are as patient-controlled as Type 1 diabetes and as patient-solvable as Type 2 diabetes. That's why it's so important for you and your loved ones to understand this disease. If you're a newly diagnosed diabetic, don't view the diagnosis as a sentence to a shorter life but as an opportunity to live a longer, healthier, more enjoyable life.

Your Doctor Can Guide You but You're in Control

Your doctor can diagnose, explain, and get you on the right path but he or she isn't living with diabetes daily like you are. By reading this book and applying what you learn, you'll be on your way to a healthier life from the first day you open it and within two months you can normalize your blood sugars, feel better, and look better.

What You'll Learn

By testing my blood sugars six, eight, or even 10 or more times a day for more than 35 years*, I've learned what foods require the least amount of insulin and therefore contribute to weight loss and lower blood sugars. Conversely, I've learned what foods trigger the most insulin demand and therefore are the biggest contributors to weight gain and blood sugar increases. It's taken me more than 35 years to learn which foods to maximize, which foods to moderate, and which foods to minimize.

You will learn which foods to eat and when to eat them in a few days by reading and understanding this book.

➠ You'll also understand the simple science of weight loss.

*AUTHOR'S NOTE:

I refer to having diabetes for over 50 years, but I refer to about 35 years of learning about foods. The reason for the difference is that for my first 15 to 16 years as a diabetic no self-testing was available. In those years, I learned very little about what foods were good for diabetics and what foods weren't. It was the advent of self-testing in the early 1980s that gave me the tool to understand the impact of foods on blood sugar, health, and weight.

➠ You'll understand why insulin is called the "traffic stop-and-go light" of weight loss and weight gain.

➠ You'll know which foods will overwork your pancreas and prevent it from being able to produce enough insulin to normalize your blood sugars.

➠ You'll know which foods will give your pancreas the relief it needs to produce sufficient insulin to normalize your blood sugars.

➠ You'll know how it feels to be free of the fear of the severe complications that face Type 2 diabetics.

➠ And finally, you'll know how it feels to be healthy again.

Activity and Exercise

Is your eating lifestyle the whole story? No. Activity and exercise also play a role. But what you put into your body is by far and away more important than how you burn it. I'll explain and defend that statement later in this book.

Activity and exercise are important to good health, good appearance, and healthy longevity. By testing my blood sugar regularly after activities and after exercising, I have learned what kind of exercises and activities are best, how much you should be doing to most effectively control your blood sugar and your weight. You'll also learn why it's important to toss the old, discouraging exercise adage of "no pain, no gain" into the trash can of bad advice.

Don't cringe when I say exercise. This is not a serious bodybuilding regimen, it's a program for people 40 and older or for those who may never have been in a health club or gym and who aren't as active as they used to be. You'll learn how simple changes in your activity and exercise patterns will change your life. These simple, smart lifestyle changes will improve your health, your appearance, your outlook, and your longevity.

The *Diabetes Lifeline Diet*™

In this book you'll be introduced to the *Diabetes Lifeline Diet*™. This is not a diet in the conventional sense with a set time to lose weight and then return to your existing eating habits. It's an *eating lifestyle* that will result in changes in your eating patterns until those patterns become habits that you follow without struggle or thought. Those new habits will be easy for you to maintain and enjoy the rest of your healthier life.

Knowing the impact of the foods you eat on your blood sugar level is so very important, not only for Type 2 diabetics but also for pre-diabetics, borderline diabetics, and anyone who wants to lose weight. Eating the wrong foods will raise your blood sugar too fast and too much and result in significant weight gain. Conversely, eating the right foods will reduce blood sugar, reduce insulin demand, and reduce your weight.

For Type 2 diabetics—when embracing the advice in this book you will likely eliminate all your symptoms of diabetes. Some may call that curing your Type 2 diabetes, others may call it reversing Type 2 diabetes but whatever you call it, you will reduce or eliminate the devastating complications of diabetes. You will feel better, look better, be slimmer, and be healthier. This book is your jump start to that healthier life.

Chapter 1

Diabetes Simplified

Understanding Type 2 Diabetes from a Patient's Point of View

Understanding diabetes starts with understanding how the food you eat is converted to energy for your body to use in everyday activities. Most descriptions of diabetes are, of course, written by researchers or doctors, many of whom have in-depth knowledge of the body's chemistry, structural biology, and physiology. To be as precise as pos-sible, many of their descriptions get too complicated for the typical diabetic, especially a newly diagnosed diabetic to understand. It's my goal to be as clear and understandable as possible as I try to give each of you the knowledge you need to deal with Type 2 diabetes, border-line diabetes, prediabetes, and weight loss.

AUTHOR'S NOTE:

Throughout this book, the language is simple and straightforward, designed to promote your under-standing of diabetes to help you make your own good decisions.

As a 53-year Type 1 diabetic, I've spent the last 35 years—since self-testing has been available—working to understand the impact of food and activity on blood sugar and weight. For three years, I structured my research, created detailed charts of the impact of foods and combinations of foods, and graphed the results. This testing brings a unique, never-before-done answer to America's commonly asked health question: "What should I eat to reverse or avoid Type 2 diabetes?

What Happens When a Nondiabetic Eats or Drinks for Energy and Nourishment?

The best way to understand diabetes is to first understand what happens when a *nondiabetic* eats food and converts it to energy.

When a nondiabetic eats food *all* that food is converted to some amount of glucose. Some foods convert to *large amounts* of glucose, other foods to *small amounts* of glucose. Some foods enter the bloodstream as glucose quickly. Other foods enter the bloodstream as glucose more slowly.

When glucose starts entering the bloodstream it triggers a rise in what is commonly referred to as blood sugar or blood glucose. As the blood sugar begins to rise, a signal is sent to the pancreas to start producing insulin, which is a hormone that allows the glucose that goes into the bloodstream to be absorbed through walls of the bloodstream into the body's cells for energy and storage. In a nondiabetic, the pancreas obliges and produces just the right amount of insulin.

That insulin also allows the excess glucose that isn't used for energy to be stored as fat. That's a very important point to remember. Glucose that you don't need for energy gets stored as fat—first in the liver and then around the body in all the places where you don't want it.

The more glucose you allow into your bloodstream, the less likely you are to use it all, allowing the excess to be stored as fat.

In a nondiabetic, when sufficient insulin has been produced to allow the body to use or store the glucose in the bloodstream and the level of glucose in the bloodstream returns to normal levels, the pancreas stops sending any more insulin to the bloodstream and the blood sugar stabilizes at that normal* level.

Think of it this way. For a non-diabetic, eating is like heating a house in the winter using a thermostat. When the house gets too cold, the thermostat sends a message to the furnace that says, "Turn on the heat." When the furnace brings the heat up to the set (normal) temperature, the thermostat sends the signal to stop sending up heat. That's the way things are supposed to work. But what if the pancreas doesn't produce enough insulin? That's the challenge Type 2 diabetics have and borderline, or pre-diabetics, will have if they don't take preventive action.

Before we get to Type 2 diabetes, it will help you to understand Type 1 diabetes.

*AUTHOR'S NOTE:

Normal level is generally considered to be between 75 and 105 mg/dl (that's milligrams of sugar (glucose) per deciliter of blood). You don't need to remember the "milligrams per deciliter" part but you do need to know the term, blood sugar and what the normal, healthy level is.

What Happens When a Type 1 Diabetic Eats or Drinks for Energy and Nourishment

Now we know what happens when a nondiabetic eats (or drinks), but what happens when an *untreated* Type 1 diabetic eats food? Well, it's the same as for a nondiabetic—*up to a point.*

When a Type 1 diabetic eats food, some of that food is converted to glucose and absorbed through the stomach lining and into the bloodstream just as it is with a nondiabetic. When the glucose starts entering the bloodstream it triggers a rise in blood sugar just as it does in a nondiabetic. As the blood sugar begins to rise, the pancreas gets a signal to start producing insulin so the body can use or store the energy the blood sugar will provide.

This is where things change. The pancreas says, "Sorry, I don't do that." If no insulin is produced or if no insulin is injected with a syringe or infused with an insulin pump, the glucose can't get out of the bloodstream into the cells to provide energy to live. Without insulin, the Type 1 diabetic will die within a very short period of time.

Prior to the discovery of insulin, the life expectancy of Type 1 diabetics was short indeed. Typically, they lived for just months after diagnosis and during that time they were so weak and so sick that they couldn't perform routine life activities. The discovery of insulin in the early 1920s by Dr. Frederick Banting and Charles Best, working at the University of Toronto, changed the life expectancy for Type 1 diabetics from just months to multiple decades and changed the quality and functionality of Type 1 diabetics' lives dramatically.

Now, What Happens When a Type 2 Diabetic Eats or Drinks for Energy and Nourishment?

The process for a Type 2 diabetic is also the same as for a nondiabetic and Type 1 diabetic—up to a point.

When a Type 2 diabetic eats food, some of that food is absorbed through the stomach walls and enters into the bloodstream as glucose just as it does with a nondiabetic and a Type 1 diabetic. When the glucose starts entering the bloodstream it triggers a rise in blood sugar. As the blood sugar begins to rise, the pancreas gets a signal to start producing insulin.

This is where things change. In a Type 2 diabetic the pancreas says, *"I've been working too hard trying to produce the insulin needed for all the glucose you've been creating. I'm tired and I can't produce all the insulin you need. But I will produce what I can and hope it helps."* Implicit in this message is that if the Type 2 diabetic will reduce the amount of glucose in the bloodstream, it will reduce the demand for insulin and the pancreas will be able to produce sufficient insulin to meet that demand.

This is essentially the difference between Type 1 and Type 2 diabetes. In a Type 1 diabetic, no insulin is produced. In a Type 2 diabetic the pancreas is producing some insulin but not enough to get all the glucose out of the bloodstream and into the cells that need the glucose for energy, nourishment, and storage.

The result is that blood sugar is often above normal and it's that higher-than-normal blood sugar that causes the terrible complications that are described in the next chapter. But you'll learn in subsequent chapters that Type 2 diabetes is avoidable and reversible.

This insufficiency of insulin is most commonly related to eating too much of the wrong foods combined with a relatively sedentary lifestyle, and increasing age. Most likely it's some combination of these characteristics, but getting older and heavier is the most common journey to Type 2 diabetes. We can't do much about getting older; in fact, that's better than the alternative. But this book will show you exactly how to ease the burden on your pancreas and lose weight.

Characteristics of Type 2 Diabetes Compared to Type 1 Diabetes

Type 2 diabetes is much slower to develop than Type 1 and is much subtler. It may be present for years before it is discovered.

Type 2 diabetics can sometimes be treated with oral medications that eliminate the symptoms and some Type 2 diabetics may need insulin injections to supplement the insulin their bodies are producing. But the very best and healthiest way to deal with Type 2 diabetes is to eat the right foods.

The best news of all for Type 2 diabetics is that most can eliminate all the symptoms of diabetes and rid themselves of the need to take any medication just by adjusting their eating lifestyle.

Some doctors will call this a cure for Type 2 diabetes and some will say that's just eliminating the symptoms. Whichever is correct, the end result is that your body will act just like a healthy nondiabetic's, and that means a longer, healthier, and likely happier life—and that's a very good thing.

Type 2 diabetes is usually contracted later in life than Type 1 diabetes. Type 1 diabetics are typically—but not always— diagnosed between birth and their late 20s and the onset is not related to lifestyle habits or weight.

Type 2 diabetics are most often diagnosed from their 40s on. The onset is very often— but again not always— related primarily to less-than-healthy eating habits. Because they are typically older than Type 1s when they are diagnosed, Type 2 diabetics have a shorter time than Type 1 diabetics to accept the diagnosis and create the new lifestyle necessary for a long, healthy life.

Are Type 2 Diabetics "Insulin-Dependent" or "Insulin-Assisted?"

In the early stages of medical distinction between the two types of diabetes, I wish the term used to describe Type 2 diabetics who use insulin had been established as *insulin-assisted*, not *insulin-dependent*. As a Type 2 diabetic you may need that insulin assistance now but if you can make some key changes in your eating lifestyle, you won't need that assistance from either insulin or oral medication in the future. This book will show you what changes you need to make and how to make those changes.

Pre-diabetics, Borderline Diabetics, and All Overweight People

In addition to Type 2 diabetics and borderline diabetics, the third group of people who will benefit greatly from the information in this book are those folks who are overweight. Even though you may have no symptoms of diabetes, you are much more likely to get diabetes than those who are not overweight. Although a number of issues influence the likelihood of getting Type 2 diabetes, no one characteristic is more closely related to Type 2 diabetes than excessive weight.

The most common estimate is that about 80 percent of Type 2 diabetics are overweight or obese. When you combine that statistic with the Center for Disease Control's estimate that about one third of Americans are obese and another one third are just overweight, you can understand the huge increases in Type 2 diabetes. (See graph on following page).

As you review the dramatic increases in diabetes in the United States as shown in this graph, make note of the fact that 1980 witnessed the creation of the Food Pyramid and by 1990 the Food Pyramid had changed America's eating habits. Those new eating habits marked the beginning of the obesity and Type 2 diabetes epidemic in the United States. A more recent report from the *National Diabetes Statistics Report* 2014 indicated the number of Type 2 diabetics in the United States at that time was close to 30 million.

NUMBER (*in Millions*) OF PEOPLE WITH DIAGNOSED TYPE 2 DIABETES IN THE UNITED STATES, 1980–2011

The incidence of diabetes has increased dramatically in the United States since the inception of the Food Pyramid in 1980.

The 2014 estimate of the number of Type 2 diabetics in the United States is about 30 million.

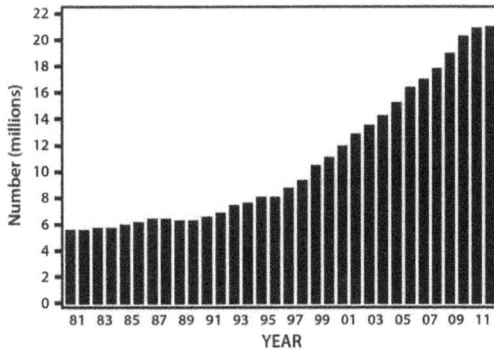

To cure or reverse Type 2 diabetes, to assure your long-term good health, to lose weight, or to avoid getting Type 2 diabetes in the first place, you need an understanding of the disease, a desire to be healthy, a positive attitude, and knowledge of what foods you should be eating. Subsequent chapters will give you an understanding of foods that will be life-changing. But before we get to that information, I need to provide a little more motivation for you to make healthy changes. This next chapter will highlight some problems you may face if you don't keep your blood sugar and weight under control.

Chapter 2

The Dangers of High Blood Sugars and Type 2 Diabetes

Your Blood Sugar Is High but You *Feel* Okay.

What's the Problem?

Over and over I hear the same quiet and melancholy reflections from middle-aged and older Type 2 diabetics who may be suffering from circulatory problems, kidney failure, serious vision problems, foot sores, or foot ulcers, "I should have taken my high blood sugars more seriously." Or "I wish I had been more conscientious about my blood sugars years ago." It's sad to hear those comments but they are very understandable.

Why are High Blood Sugars Easy to Ignore?

Based on my experience and hundreds of conversations with Type 2 diabetics, I've learned the biggest reason diabetics often let blood sugar levels drift high—and remain high—is the lack of immediate negative feedback from their bodies. If your blood sugar gets too low, you know it. I mean right away. You're in danger and you better do something—right now.

But high blood sugars are more subtle than low blood sugars and can be harder to identify until they reach a very high and very unhealthy point. With normal considered in the 75–105 mg/dl range, what happens when your blood sugar gets up to 120? What do you feel? *Nothing*.

How about 140? Still *nothing*. What about 160? 180? You still feel normal. How can you be sick if you feel normal?

Maybe at 200 mg/dl or higher you might feel just a little off. You can't put your finger on it but you don't feel great. By the time your blood sugar gets to 300, you usually can feel it. It feels like you might be getting the flu. You're not sick but you feel just a little under the weather. Even then, you're in no *immediate* danger so you'll tend to not treat it as seriously as you should.

Why Is it So Important to Take High Blood Sugars Seriously?

As a key part of your background, you need to understand what is likely to happen if you are careless or indifferent in your blood sugar control. And you need to know why so many diabetics regret their inattention or indifference to high blood sugars years later. I cover those dangers in detail in this chapter.

This is going to be a pretty frightening chapter to read but remember that all the serious consequences I talk about can be avoided. If you're already experiencing some of these problems, their progression can be slowed, and many can even be reversed.

How Long Are "Long-Term" Problems?

When I talk about the consequences of long-term high blood sugar, what do I mean? *Long-term* is totally dependent on the age and physical condition of a diabetic when he or she is diagnosed. For example, it stands to reason that a newly diagnosed young diabetic is starting his or her life as a diabetic—likely Type 1— with a healthier circulatory system, healthier kidneys, and a healthier heart than a newly diagnosed 60-year-old Type 2 diabetic.

What that means is that the young person has more time to learn about dealing with diabetes and to develop the habits he or she needs to live a long and healthy life. It's better for the young person to learn quickly but a slower adaptation is likely going to be less damaging to a younger diabetic than to an older diabetic.

Older Diabetics Must Act Quickly

The older Type 2 diabetic, whether insulin-dependent or not, does not have the luxury of taking a lot of time to change habits. A few years of high blood sugars for someone in their 40s, 50s, 60s, 70s, or 80s can have a very negative impact on health and survivability whereas a few years of higher-than-ideal blood sugars for a younger person will not have as significant an impact.

This is a problem that must be taken seriously by people diagnosed with diabetes later in life. If you're diagnosed with Type 2 diabetes (insulin-dependent or not), you don't have the luxury of years before you need to start changing your habits. You need to begin acting now.

In future chapters I spend a lot of time talking about eating patterns and habits. You will be amazed and pleased at both the immediate and lifelong impact of changing your food choices. And when that change is combined with a modest but consistent exercise pattern and a slightly more active lifestyle, you're on your way to a healthier life immediately.

The Problems You Want to Avoid

Although there is no *immediate* danger in periodic high blood sugars, there certainly are very severe long-term consequences of frequent high blood sugars over extended time. Consistent high blood sugars will contribute directly to circulatory problems—which in the long term will lead to heart problems, kidney problems, vision impairment, and even blindness.

High blood sugars will also cause loss of feeling in your feet (neuropathy). This loss of feeling in your feet means you won't feel punctures, lacerations, abrasions, or blisters in your feet, which untreated or unhealed can lead to amputation of toes, feet, or even legs.

The 9-Year Diabetic Control and Complications Study

The comprehensive nine-year *Diabetic Control and Complications Trial* (often referred to as the DCCT study) established conclusively that *"for all diabetics the better their control the less likely they are to have complications and the worse their control, the more likely they are to have complications."* Five years later, the *United Kingdom Prospective Diabetes Study* re-confirmed that good blood sugar control will prevent complications. These complications are universally referred to as "diabetic complications" and should be a part of your regular discussions with your doctor.

Now let's get into some specifics so you understand why high blood sugar causes these problems and why it's so important for you to work to prevent these problems from occurring.

1. Vision Impairment and Blindness

The diabetic vision issues generally referred to as *retinopathy* are caused by clogging of the tiny blood capillaries in the eye. These micro-vessels get partially blocked and form what are called aneurisms. *Aneurisms* are bulges in those tiny capillaries that may sometimes burst. If they do burst and if the blood blocks the macula portion of the eye, vision is instantly impaired. In most cases burst aneurisms can be treated by laser but in many cases an still cause significant vision loss.

In the early '80s when I was 37 or 38, my doctor, Jeanne Bonar, wanted me to start biannual visits to an ophthalmologist. She explained that this was important in tracking the success or lack of success of my diabetic control.

She explained that the tiny capillaries in the retina are the only blood vessels in the body that are externally visible. These capillaries are a window to your diabetic health. Problems with those capillaries indicate that you likely have other circulatory problems and need to improve your blood sugar control. Problem-free capillaries indicate that you're doing well with your control.

My first visit with Dr. Swanson, an ophthalmologist in Anchorage, was in late 1981 or early 1982. He discovered what he called background retinopathy. He explained that I had some small aneurisms in both eyes. They were quite minor and not an immediate worry. But if they got worse, the capillaries could burst and cause a blockage of the macula, which could impair my vision.

For the past 10 years, my current ophthalmologist, Dr. Griff Steiner, has monitored my eyes. During a biannual eye exam in 2011, he told me the aneurisms had gradually disappeared in one eye and diminished to the point of near disappearance in the other eye. When he finished his exam, he stood up, smiled, and said, "I can hardly tell you have diabetes." That was one of those simple, straightforward statements that I'll never forget, especially after having had diabetes for over 47 years at that time. During my last visit in 2013, Dr. Steiner told me that my aneurisms had completely disappeared in both eyes. The lesson here is that some diabetic complications can be reversed.

I'm convinced that regular visits to an ophthalmologist will open a clear and helpful window into your health as a diabetic and whether your visits result in a positive report or not, I believe that when you leave the office you'll be inspired to keep working on good or better blood sugar control.

You should ask your doctor if you should be seeing an ophthalmologist.

2. Foot Problems: Neuropathy and Angiopathy

Neuropathy, as I mentioned earlier, is a loss of feeling in the extremities, most often in the feet. The danger here is the potential for blisters and small injuries to the feet to go unnoticed and become serious problems before they are addressed.

A common complication of poorly controlled diabetes is impaired circulation, which often manifests itself in the feet first. Injuries or blisters that may occur in your feet—while you can't feel their onset—are complicated by the fact that poor long-term diabetic care also results in limited circulation in your feet. That makes healing much more difficult and injuries to your feet much more serious.

This is a more significant problem for longer-term, older diabetics than it is for younger diabetics, since circulation is naturally diminished as a function of age. These foot problems are typically exacerbated by the length of time a person has poorly controlled diabetes.

It's very important for older or longer-term diabetics to establish a relationship with a podiatrist. I've done that and have learned a lot about foot problems and care from Dr. Ken Swayman, an Anchorage podiatrist. Dr. Swayman is an excellent communicator, who has helped me immensely with a toe problem that provides a perfect illustration of what can happen when diabetes-caused neuropathy comes into play.

The only complication I have so far from diabetes after over 50 years is a moderate loss of feeling in my feet (neuropathy). This neuropathy has caused me a few problems in the past dozen or so years.

Not only are foot problems the most frequent cause of hospitalization among diabetics, but also, diabetes is the biggest cause of amputations in the United States. Over 100,000 diabetes-related amputations of toes, feet, or legs were performed last year alone and many started with toe lacerations, abrasions, or blisters.

My Suggestions for Diabetic Foot Care

To avoid blisters—which I may not feel—I use well-broken-in, comfortable golf shoes and tend to stick with the brand of tennis or athletic shoes that have proven to be friends of my feet. My current choice of brands for my athletic shoes is *Brooks* and *Salomon*—both very comfortable and supportive. My choice for golf shoes is *Footjoy*. For dress shoes, I've found that *Dr. Comfort* shoes are also very comfortable and have not caused any blisters. I have recently discovered Skechers shoes and have found them to be extremely comfortable, supportive and adaptive to my foot.

If you already have loss of feeling in your feet, I suggest you buy some thin white cotton or nylon socks to wear under your normal socks. That will not only provide a better cushion for your feet and help prevent blisters but the white under-socks will also make it easy to spot any bleeding from blisters that you may not feel.

I also encourage you to put *Cetaphil* moisturizing cream on your feet regularly and keep a hand mirror in your nightstand so you can check your feet for injuries that you may not feel. But an even better solution is to maintain good blood sugar control and not give sensory or circulatory problems a foothold.

**Good Foot Care Is Very Important
for Middle-Aged and Older Diabetics**

If you're a middle-aged or older diabetic, your feet deserve attention. If blood sugars are too high, your feet may very well be the first indicator that you need to improve your blood sugar control. You should be asking your doctor if he or she thinks you should start seeing a podiatrist. You'll learn a lot and likely postpone or completely avoid some serious problems.

Neuropathy is not necessarily a precursor to amputation. Most long-term or older diabetics will develop some neuropathy but only a small minority will require amputation. That's a minority you don't want to be a part of.

3. Kidney Disease

Kidney disease is another potential problem with diabetes that can be avoided with good blood sugar control. Fortunately, I don't have any personal experience with kidney disease, but I do have a basic understanding of the kidney function and do have friends who have died because of diabetes-related kidney failure.

In everyday language, the role of kidneys is to filter waste products out of the bloodstream and into the urine for elimination from the body. When the kidneys stop working properly, some products from the blood, such as protein, start showing up in the urine. This is usually the first indication of kidney problems. At this early stage there are typically no other noticeable symptoms.

The kidneys are also responsible for maintaining a balance between water and salt in your bloodstream. When the kidneys are not functioning properly, an imbalance can occur which will often create a significant rise in blood pressure.

Like other diabetic complications, this has a direct relationship to blood sugar. My friend and golfing buddy, Dr. Rob Benedetti, formerly medical director and a kidney specialist at the Rockwood Clinic in Spokane, says the most common causes of kidney problems are high blood sugar, high blood pressure, and excessive doses of over-the-counter pain medication.

The better your blood sugar control, the less likely it is that kidney problems will occur. The more consistently high your blood sugar is, the more likely you will experience kidney problems. You should ask your doctor about periodic urine tests to determine if any early indication of kidney disease is present.

An excellent and more detailed explanation of diabetic kidney disease is contained in *The Johns Hopkins Guide to Diabetes* by Christopher D. Saudek, M.D., Richard R. Rubin, Ph.D., and Cynthia S. Shump, R.N., pages 310-313.

4. Arteriosclerosis and Heart Disease

The heart, the brain, the eyes, and the legs can all be affected by arteriosclerosis. It can be caused by—among other things—poorly controlled diabetes.

The dramatic increase in Type 2 diabetes coincides very closely with the introduction of the Food Pyramid in 1980. *Our Government's message—promoted through the Food Pyramid—has been if you don't want to get fat, don't eat fat; if you don't want heart problems, don't eat fat; if you don't want circulatory problems, don't eat fat; and if you don't want to get Type 2 diabetes, don't eat fat; but do eat 6-11 helpings of grain and wheat products.*

The Problem is the Government was Wrong!

Over the past 35-plus years, since self-testing has been available, I've gradually increased the amount of butter I've eaten. I've increased my butter consumption for two reasons: first, it dramatically improves the taste of vegetables so I eat more of these healthy foods and second, butter does not raise my blood sugar much.

What I do know for certain based on my 60,000 self-administered blood sugar tests is that eating butter does not result in measurable increases in blood sugars or in weight gain. But in terms of heart disease, cholesterol, and arteriosclerosis, I must rely on others' research.

What Others Say!

On June 23, 2014, *Time Magazine's* cover headlined the words **"Eat Butter."** The subhead declared **"Scientists labeled fat the enemy. Why they were wrong."**

The New York Times on February 19, 2015 said "…major health groups like the American Heart Association in recent years have backed away from dietary cholesterol restrictions" …

Runner's World Magazine in their January/February 2015 edition in a story titled "Eat Fat, Be Fit" led the story as follows:

> *"Runners like to follow the rules. And for decades, nutrition rules put a strict limit on saturated fat. After all, as far back as the 1960s, experts have decreed that eating foods high in saturated fat such as eggs, red meat, and full-fat dairy, will increase your risk of heart disease. So runners took heed, all but banishing those foods from their diets.*
>
> *But a string of news-making studies has flipped that idea on its head. One of those headline-catchers published in the Annals of Internal Medicine early last year, reviewed 76 existing studies and found no association between saturated fat and heart disease. The new emerging thought (is): 'Saturated fat may not be the demon that it was made out to be,' says Jeff Volek, Ph.D., R.D., associate professor in the department of kinesiology at the University of Connecticut."*

I've become more aligned in my thinking with the growing number of researchers and doctors who no longer believe fat is the villain it has been made out to be.

In the words of Dr. John Mues, an internal medicine specialist, a friend of mine, and a well-conditioned 67-year-old athlete, **"Fat is your friend."**

Conclusion: Avoiding These Deadly Complications

As you read these complications as a package, they can be very scary. But remember this: *These complications are all avoidable.* If you already have one or more of these complications, the negative impact of the complication(s) can in most cases be dramatically slowed and in some cases reversed by making changes based on recommendations in this book.

Glucose Testing

In my opinion, the most valuable tools for diabetes control are blood glucose testers. The availability of these testers and the ease and quickness of being able to test blood sugars are, I believe, among the biggest advancements in helping all diabetics and pre-diabetics achieve long-term health. Blood sugar testing will help insulin-dependent Type 2 diabetics learn how to balance the three factors that control blood sugar: food, insulin, and exercise. For all diabetics, testing will confirm what you'll learn in this book and teach you over time what foods cause the greatest rise in your blood sugar and the greatest weight gains and what foods do not.

In the balance of this book, you're going to learn how to reduce or eliminate all these potential problems, and if you diligently put into practice what you'll learn you will eliminate Type 2 diabetes altogether. If you don't have diabetes, you're going to learn how to reduce your chances of ever getting it by losing weight.

Let's Get Started

By the time you finish this book, you'll have the information to live healthier, happier, and longer. You can do it.

Chapter 3

The Simple Science of Reversing Type 2 Diabetes and Losing Weight

For Type 2 Diabetics, Borderline Diabetics, and Pre-diabetics and Any Overweight Person Who Wants to Lose Weight

Understand and Remember This:

1. You can't win in a fight against hunger.

2. You can't lose weight by cutting way back on eating and being hungry all the time.

3. You can lose weight by eating more of the right foods and less of the wrong foods.

4. Which foods are right and which are wrong?

The answer is in this book.

This chapter provides the essential background for Type 2 diabetics to understand how to lower blood sugar, lose weight, eliminate the symptoms, and avoid the complications of Type 2 diabetes. It will teach pre-diabetics or borderline diabetics how to avoid ever getting Type 2 diabetes. This chapter will also show nondiabetics how to lose weight and avoid ever getting diabetes.

The best action *Type 2 diabetics, pre-diabetics, or borderline diabetics* can take to avoid diabetic complications and eliminate the need to take medications or injections is to first lower their blood sugars. When you change your eating patterns to lower your blood sugar, your weight will start coming off. When those eating patterns become habits your weight will stay off. The result will be a healthier, happier, longer life.

By the time you finish this chapter, you'll have the information and understanding you need to lower your blood sugars and start losing weight. But more important, you'll learn how to stay at that new lower weight and maintain normal blood sugars for the rest of your life.

For most Type 2 diabetics, avoiding or eliminating the need for insulin injections is a high priority and evidence of dietary success.

By following the path provided by this book, the vast majority of Type 2 diabetics will be able to avoid or eliminate the need for insulin injections or oral medications.

Weight Gain and the Type 2 Diabetic Epidemic

The most commonly used estimate of the number of Type 2 diabetics in the United States is 30 million, compared to about 3 million Type 1 diabetics. Many argue that the rate of increase of Type 2 diabetes puts it in the category of an epidemic, although unlike other more infamous epidemics such as the bubonic plague, influenza, cholera, and smallpox, it doesn't pose the likelihood of immediate death. It does, however, pose the likelihood of a significantly shortened and unhealthy lifespan.

Not only will unchecked Type 2 diabetes significantly shorten life span, but the precursors to diabetes, "prediabetes" and "borderline diabetes," may have already started the life-shortening process. High blood pressure and heart disease may also already be evident.

How important is weight in this epidemic? First, not all Type 2 diabetics are overweight and not all overweight people have Type 2 diabetes. Type 2 diabetes may in some cases be hereditary and may in some cases be culturally influenced, *but without question the most common characteristic associated with Type 2 diabetics is being overweight.*

Consequently, losing weight is the very best action you can take to lower your blood sugar. Almost all Type 2 diabetics would like to lose weight. But that is much easier said than done. How can we change that?

America's Weight Loss Strategy Has Been Backwards

As a Type 2 diabetic, pre-diabetic, or borderline diabetic you've probably read books or pamphlets in which the authors suggest losing weight in order to lower your blood sugar. That's fair and that's a good recommendation. But then they are likely to say, "If you lose weight, your blood sugars will go down." That is not an incorrect statement but in terms of function *it's backward.* What they should be saying is, "If you bring your blood sugars down you *will lose weight.*"

Key Point
Why has weight loss been so hard for Type 2 diabetics?

The answer is simple:
America has been going about it the wrong way.

What's the Difference?
And Why is that Difference so Important?

First, it's very, very difficult to lose weight unless you focus on bringing your blood sugars down first. That's why so many weight loss programs and diets fail. Second, by lowering your blood sugars you are attacking the very source of the problem that has contributed to your weight gain; and third, the sooner you lower your blood sugars the less likely you are to suffer debilitating diabetic complications.

Don't try to lose weight in order to lower your blood sugars. First work to lower your blood sugars, then *you will lose weight.*

Keeping in mind the goal of lowering your blood sugars to normal levels to avoid diabetic complications and lose weight, the next logical question is how you do that.

You need to start by understanding how we gain and lose weight.

Understanding How We Gain or Lose Weight

The decision maker in weight gain or loss is *insulin*. It has often been called "nature's 'fat' traffic light" because it directs and facilitates the glucose in your bloodstream to be used either for energy, for short-term storage in and around your liver as glycogen, or for long-term storage around your body as fat. That storage around your body is the fat that's hardest to get rid of. But you'll understand how to get rid of that fat by the end of this chapter.

In everyday language, here's how insulin determines whether or not you will get fat. When you eat a meal that includes say, protein, fat, and any type of carbohydrates—I'll explain later how I categorize carbohydrates—all of that food will be converted to some amount of glucose and show up in your bloodstream as blood glucose.

Some foods will turn into a lot of glucose and other foods will turn into just a little glucose. Learning which is which is your key to lower blood sugars, weight loss, and a healthier life.

What Determines How Much Glucose is Used as Energy and How Much is Stored as Fat?

That determination is largely a function of *how much* glucose is entering your bloodstream and *how fast* it's entering.

If more glucose is going into your bloodstream than is needed to provide energy for your daily activities, the remainder will be stored. As you now know, your body's first choice for storage—after its energy need is filled—is in the liver as glycogen. That glycogen will become a readily available source of energy in case you don't eat again for a few hours. The next choice for storage—after the liver storage is fulfilled—is around your body as body fat.

That's How Energy is Stored Now How is it Used?

The choices for your body's usage of the glucose in your bloodstream created by the food you eat, will always follow the same pattern. Your body will always choose the easiest source of energy first. That means the available glucose in your bloodstream will always be the first to be used. If you need more energy than the available glucose will provide, your body will tap its second choice—glycogen from the liver, which is also easily returned to your bloodstream for use as energy. Only when both of those choices are insufficient will your body call on its third choice—fat stored in and around your organs and body.

So How Do You Lose the Fat Stored Around Your Body?

You now know that the fat stored in and around your organs and body will be used for energy *only* when the other two sources—glucose in your bloodstream and glycogen in your liver—are depleted. So to lose body fat you need to put less glucose in your bloodstream so your body will automatically begin using the fat in your liver and then the fat around your body. Your body will use that fat automatically if you put less glucose in your bloodstream.

Key Points

1. Losing weight doesn't mean eating less food and always being hungry. It means eating less of the food that puts lots of glucose in your bloodstream and more of the food that doesn't put a lot of glucose in your bloodstream.

2. Remember I said to lose weight you must first lower your blood sugar.

How Will You Know What Foods will Put the Least Amount of Glucose in Your Bloodstream?

The answer to that question is what this book is all about. Keep reading.

Another Benefit of Less Glucose in Your Blood

When you decrease the amount of glucose in your bloodstream you also decrease the amount of insulin that your pancreas must produce; in other words, your over-worked pancreas gets a breather and doesn't have to work as hard.

Conversely, when you increase the amount of glucose going into your bloodstream you also increase the amount of insulin that your pancreas must produce; in other words, your already overworked pancreas will have to work harder.

So now you're beginning to understand why the amount of glucose created by different foods is important to you.

Key Point

I would not be overstating if I were to say to all diabetics, pre-diabetics, or borderline diabetics that lowering your blood glucose levels and committing to keeping those levels normal is going to make the difference between living **a long, healthy life and a short, unhealthy life.**

Summary of the Benefits of Lowering Blood Sugars

Lowering the amount of glucose entering your bloodstream will give you four very important results:

First, less glucose in your bloodstream means your body will use glycogen from your liver and then use the fat you have stored around your body, which will result in weight loss.

Second, less glucose in your bloodstream means your pancreas will produce less insulin; and less insulin means less new fat storage.

Third, your overworked pancreas will be able to produce enough insulin to normalize your glucose.

And *fourth,* by keeping your glucose normal, you can postpone or avoid completely all the devastating complications from high blood sugar and poorly controlled diabetes.

Conclusion

Excess glucose is the cause and creator of fat and the cause of Type 2 diabetes.

When you get—and keep—your blood sugars down to normal levels you will have reversed or avoided Type 2 diabetes.

Insulin may be the "fat decision maker" but too much glucose is the villain. Periodically I'll see authors referring to too much insulin as the cause of weight gain; but insulin is just the responder to too much glucose.

How Much Glucose You Create Is Critical but Another Important Issue is How *Fast* That Glucose Gets into Your Bloodstream

How much glucose you put into your bloodstream is a major factor in weight gain and getting Type 2 diabetes. But *how fast* different foods cause your blood sugar levels to rise is also very important.

Some foods convert to glucose much faster than others. If the foods you eat cause your blood glucose to rise *faster* than you can burn it, the remainder will be stored in the liver as glycogen or around your body as fat. Foods that enter your bloodstream as glucose *more slowly* allow you to use more of that glucose before it gets stored.

It's important for all diabetics to understand it's not only about the blood glucose *increase* that a given food or combination of foods cause, but also the *speed* of that increase.

Both the size of the blood sugar increase and the speed of that increase are contributors to weight gain and Type 2 diabetes.

How Do I Know This?

As a Type 1 diabetic I use an insulin pump. It's my only source of insulin. My pancreas produces no insulin on its own. This is unlike Type 2 diabetics' pancreases, which produce some insulin but just not enough for the foods they eat.

Because my pancreas produces no insulin, and if I don't use my pump to inject (or infuse) insulin, I am able to determine exactly how much each food or combination of foods raises blood sugar.

What I've Learned about Foods, Blood Sugars, and Weight Gain

Here's what I've learned over the past 35 years about the relationship between insulin and weight gain.

At the end of each day, my pump can tell me how much insulin I've pumped in that day. If what I've eaten over a period of a week produces an amount of glucose that requires me to give myself an average of about 34 units a day of insulin, I will gain weight during that week.

If the food I've eaten over a week requires me to give myself an average of about 26 units of insulin a day, I will lose weight during that week.

If my insulin requirement averages 30 units of insulin a day for a week, I neither gain nor lose weight.

These examples presume that my activity and exercise are constant. If I exercise more or less in a given week that will have an impact on weight gain or loss—but not nearly as much as the food that I eat. (More on the role of exercise and activity later in this book.)

Will the Speed and the Size of the Increases be the Same for Everyone?

In general, yes. The speed at which the foods enter the bloodstream will be for all practical purposes the same for all people. The size of the increases will vary based on the size and weight of the person.

I'm 6 feet 3 inches and weigh about 190 pounds. A person who weighs, say, 60 pounds more than I do would have a bigger volume of blood. If he or she were to eat the same foods and *same portion size* I did, his or her blood sugar would not go up as much as mine would. Much as if you put a teaspoon of sugar in an 8-ounce glass of iced tea and your friend put the same amount of sugar in a 16-ounce glass of iced tea. Both people would be impacted by the sugar at the same speed but your friend's drink would be only half as sweet.

The converse of this is true also. A smaller person—if he or she ate the same portion size of food that I did—would experience a greater rise of blood sugar.

That distinction based on body size is not critical to the message of this book. Even if you do not change the amount or portion size of the food you eat but follow my recommendations, you will ease the workload of your pancreas and you *will lose weight.*

Now if you also lower your portion size you will provide greater relief for your pancreas and you will lose more weight.

But my point is, if you reduce your insulin demand, you will lose weight—and that is true for everyone.

You now know that to reduce your insulin demand you must reduce the glucose (sugar) you put in your bloodstream.

So how do you lower your blood sugar and therefore your insulin demand?

The answer is this: You need to know what foods create lots of glucose and what foods create less glucose, which foods enter your bloodstream faster and which enter more slowly. In other words, you need to know what to eat … *and by the way, it's not what the Government has been telling us to eat for the past 35 years or so.*

How Can You Know What Foods to Eat to Reduce Work for Your Pancreas, Lower Your Blood Sugar, and Lose Weight?

The answer is, *I'm going to tell you.* That's what the core of this book reveals.

As I've previously noted, for the past 35 years I've been testing my blood sugar before and after almost every meal I've eaten. I've tested at least once—and lately twice before I go to bed each night—and after I wake up each morning. I also test before physical activities and many times after these activities. I also test at any other time I think my blood sugar needs adjusting. As a result of all these tests, I've learned how hundreds of different foods and combinations of

Key Point

It bears repeating that how much foods will raise your blood sugar and how fast foods will raise your blood sugars are both very important to your good health.

foods impact my blood sugar and weight—and will impact yours as well.

I've learned not only *how much* different foods raise my blood sugar but also *how fast* those foods raise my blood sugar—and yours as well.

What I've learned over 35 years of testing my blood sugars, you can learn in a few days by reading this book and using it as a continuing reference.

Which Foods Cause the Greatest and Fastest Rise in Blood Sugar and the Greatest Gains in Weight ... and Which Do Not

When Type 1 diabetics eat foods and cause glucose to enter the bloodstream, it cannot be used or stored naturally because no insulin is produced. The glucose simply collects in the bloodstream and causes a rise in blood sugar. This, of course, is why Type 1 diabetics need to inject the appropriate amount of insulin manually or with an insulin pump.

Only a Type 1 Diabetic Can Accurately Test the Impact of Foods on Blood Sugar

Only a Type 1 diabetic can directly and accurately test foods' impact on blood sugar. That is exactly what I've done for this book.

Although I've been testing and observing blood sugar increases for over 35 years, to derive the graphs in this book, I've specifically tested over 100 different foods or combinations of foods from all six categories and not given myself any insulin for 90 minutes. Then I've tested my blood sugar (glucose) every 10 minutes during that time to determine how much and how fast each food or combination of foods has raised my blood sugar. This will provide—never-before-published—empirical information for diabetics to lower their blood sugar and lose weight.

Why Can't Type 2 Diabetics Test Accurately to Measure the Impact of Foods on Blood Sugars?

Type 2 diabetics cannot accurately test this way since their pancreas produces some—but usually not enough—insulin and therefore even as they eat food and increase their blood sugar, their pancreas is producing some insulin and decreasing blood sugar concurrently. That partial production of insulin negates their ability to measure the exact impact of foods on their blood sugar.

When you see on my graphs that a certain food brings my blood sugar up to say 300, you, as a Type 2 diabetic, will never see your blood sugar get that high because your pancreas is producing some insulin that is bringing your blood sugar down as the food is sending it up.

What a number like 300 does tell you is that first, your pancreas has to work hard when you eat that food, and second, that your pancreas will likely not be able to bring your blood sugar down to normal, and third, you will gain weight.

Why Nondiabetics Can't Measure the Impact of Foods on Blood Sugars

Nondiabetics cannot test foods' impact on blood sugar because for them the pancreas is working properly and producing sufficient insulin to use or store their glucose automatically as it enters the bloodstream.

Consequently, their blood sugar levels never rise like a diabetic's does, and a measurement of impact of specific foods is impossible. It's important to remember that even if a nondiabetic's blood sugar doesn't show a rise, the excess glucose is still going in and being stored, so the impact on the pancreas and weight gain is still happening.

Why Hasn't This Testing and Graphing Ever Been Done Before?

We now know that only Type 1 diabetics can get an accurate measure of the impact of foods on blood glucose and less than 1 percent of America's population are Type 1 diabetics. But that's still a lot of folks, so why haven't other Type 1s done this?

First, a person who is going to do this would have to have a long history of testing and analysis to even begin. Maybe some people in the United States have tested blood sugars more than I have but I'm guessing that number is small—maybe only a handful.

I have not graphed *all* the data I gathered from 30 years of blood sugar testing. But whenever I measured, I recalled what I had most recently eaten and what activities I engaged in. After years of doing that I developed a clear understanding of the impact of different foods and food combinations. But the challenge for me in writing this book was how to represent that information graphically.

Five years ago, I started testing and measuring foods—and drinks—and graphing the results to illustrate these foods' impact on blood sugar and therefore weight.

To create these graphs, I had to be willing to make a health sacrifice—although I'm confident it's a small sacrifice. I had to be willing to eat hundreds of different foods and not take any insulin for 90 minutes. That is the only way to illustrate the impact of foods and combinations of foods on blood sugar.

I have never seen or read any information about anyone else who has actually tested the impact of foods this way. To my knowledge, this type of human testing has never been previously published or perhaps never even been done.

Researchers would be naturally hesitant to solicit diabetics to test this way because it involves the subjects' eating various foods and not taking insulin for 90 minutes—an obviously unhealthy request to make of a subject.

I did it because I believe quantifying and graphing this information and combining it with what I have learned over the past 30 years of multiple daily blood tests could help millions of diabetics have healthier, happier, longer lives.

The next chapter will show you which foods to eat and which to avoid to make lowering your blood sugar and losing weight easier than you ever dreamed possible.

Chapter 4

The New and Better Way for Diabetics to Categorize Foods

Grouping Food from a Diabetic's Perspective

This chapter provides a new look at grouping foods from a diabetic's perspective.

These groups are categorized based on *how fast* and *how much* each category of foods will raise your blood sugar. Although this book has been written primarily for diabetics to lower their blood sugar, I get more positive feedback from people who have lost weight in addition to lowering their blood sugars and A1Cs.

As you're absorbing the information in this book remember that everything I show about healthier eating, weight loss, and activity applies to nondiabetics who want to lose weight and be healthier as well as to diabetics and pre-diabetics.

The Standard Way of Describing Food Groups

From elementary school through high school and college, we've been taught the *three food groups*: proteins, fats, and carbohydrates.

Most people can name proteins—meats, fish, some vegetables, and some fats all contain some protein. And most people have some grasp of natural fats—bacon, olive oil, butter, fatty meats, and fatty fish. But ask an American to name carbohydrates and you'll get a bewildered stare and a few wild guesses.

In the standard way of looking at food groups, the best way of describing a carbohydrate is: *if it's not a protein or fat, it's a carbohydrate.* But this doesn't help you as a diabetic because you'll see in the next chapter that all natural fats act much the same in terms of impact on blood sugars and the same goes for most proteins. But carbohydrates? They're all over the board in terms of impact on blood sugars.

Carbohydrates cover a wide variety of foods that act quite differently in terms of effect on your blood sugars. For example, cauliflower is a carbohydrate and so is a bagel. Spaghetti's a carbohydrate and so is an apple. Bread is a carbohydrate and so is broccoli. Cereal is a carbohydrate and so is cabbage. Pasta's a carbohydrate and so is a grapefruit. So how can you possibly talk about carbohydrates in general because they are such a broad category and so different in their impact on blood sugar and weight?

No wonder people are confused when they are told to "eat fewer carbs." Does that mean eat less broccoli, fewer apples, less asparagus? No! When a doctor or nutritionist gives this advice they typically mean, "eat fewer starchy carbs." Starchy carbs are one of the categories that I use to clarify this carb confusion that befuddles Americans.

As of now most people are confused—understandably so—about carbs and unknowing about the impact of all foods on their blood sugar and weight.

A New and Better Way of Grouping Foods for Diabetics Based on How Much and How Fast They Raise Blood Sugar

Based on what I've learned from 35 years of testing and over 60,000 blood sugar tests, I've divided carbohydrates into four distinct groups based on how much and how fast they impact blood sugar.

This new look at food groups will help you understand what to eat and what to not eat—or more accurately what foods to eat more of and what foods to eat less of to reverse Type 2 diabetes and lose weight.

The Six Food Groups You Need to Understand

Here are the new six discrete groups of foods you need to memorize to lower your blood sugar, lose weight, and live healthier:

Sweet carbohydrates

Starchy carbohydrates

Fruit carbohydrates

Vegetable (veggie) carbohydrates

Proteins

Fats

Each of these categories of foods plays a different role in blood sugar control and weight gain. Once you understand how each category of food impacts your blood sugar and weight control, improving your health, lowering your blood sugars, and losing weight will be surprisingly easy.

The beauty of this categorization is you don't have to try to memorize how hundreds—or thousands—of foods impact your blood sugar and weight, you just need to understand how these six categories of foods impact your blood sugar and weight.

Now let's look at these categories in more detail.

More Detail on the Six Food Groups Based on Blood Sugar Impact

Sweet Carbohydrates—The Enemy Most of Us Know

Sweet carbs are made up of simple molecules—mostly lone molecules or maybe two stuck together. They're *easily dissolved and quick to enter your bloodstream*. You'll see in the graphs they are the quickest of the food categories to enter your bloodstream and will cause the greatest rise in your blood sugar. They are a big problem for diabetics and for anyone who wants to lose weight.

Once again, remember that a rise in blood sugar means more insulin demand, which means more weight gain. This is not a new revelation except in the next chapter you will see exactly how fast and how much this group will raise your blood sugar compared to other groups.

Examples of Sweet Carbohydrates

Here are examples of foods included in this category:

sugared soft drinks	ice cream sherbets and sorbets
cakes	chocolates
pies	caramels
donuts	a broad selection of desserts
sweet rolls	candy

We all know by now that too much sugar is the villain, right? Then what about all the *sugar-free* candies? Are they okay? Heck, they taste just like regular candy. But look closely at the label. You'll see that many of those items are sweetened with high-fructose corn syrup or with other sweeteners not much different from cane sugar except that they are more concentrated and make you fatter than plain cane sugar. So don't think you're doing yourself a favor by eating *sugar-free* candy. In terms of impact on blood sugar and weight, sugar-free candies often have the same and sometimes greater impact than sugared candy sweetened with cane sugar.

Both regular candy and sugar-free candy are items you need to start minimizing dramatically. This is, of course, not new information but if you do all the other things I'll propose and still eat lots of candy, you're not going to make the progress you need or want.

Many of these sweet carbohydrates will show up as sugar in your bloodstream in two to three minutes. By drinking a sugared soft drink, I can go from a low blood sugar of 50 mg/dl (milligrams of sugar per deciliter of blood) to 70 mg/dl in 90 seconds and to 120 mg/dl in three minutes. That's more than doubling the amount of sugar in my blood in three minutes.

Most of the artificial sweeteners for tea and coffee drinks do not raise blood sugars but they do encourage a continuing taste for sweet things. In addition, they include chemicals which I know nothing about. I don't use artificial sweeteners at all.

The simple sugars with no fat mixed in are the quickest to enter bloodstreams: sugared soft drinks, Skittles, jelly beans, and other candies that are pure sugar. Baked desserts such as cakes and pies usually have some fat in them, as do chocolate candy bars and ice cream. As you'll see, fat enters your bloodstream more slowly, so when fat mixes with sweet carbohydrates in your stomach, the combination is just slightly slower to enter your bloodstream than straight sweet carbohydrates, but the final impact is equal to or greater than that of pure sweets.

Take heart. In the next few chapters on actions to control blood sugar and lose weight, I'm not going to talk about cutting out desserts forever. But I will be talking about dramatically minimizing both the frequency and the quantity of desserts and sweets.

Okay. No big surprise about sweet carbs being bad in a number of ways but once you see the graphs you'll see how bad they really are.

The next category is one that will surprise quite a few people.

Starchy Carbohydrates—
The Enemy Most of Us Don't Know

These foods have a slightly more complex molecular structure than sweet carbohydrates. Their molecules are stuck together in larger strings or branching chains, which are slightly harder to break apart and are just a little bit slower to enter your bloodstream than sweets.

You'll see in the graphs that they cause a very fast and significant rise in your blood sugar, and they put a big burden on the already over-worked pancreas of a Type 2 diabetic or borderline diabetic.

Examples of Starchy Carbohydrates

Here are some examples of foods included in this category:

waffles

pancakes

dry breakfast cereals

granola

white bread of all kinds

multigrain breads (whole grain is slightly better than multigrain)

rolls

hamburger and hot dog buns

muffins

bagels

tortillas

tortilla chips

potato chips

spaghetti

lasagna

pasta

white rice (brown rice is slightly better than white rice) crackers

and other similar, starchy foods

Fruit Carbohydrates

This category has a bit of variation in how fast and how much different fruits increase blood sugar. Some fruit carbs act relatively slowly and cause moderate increases in blood sugar and weight gain and some enter the bloodstream more quickly and will cause a bigger increase in blood sugar and weight gain. This requires some distinction to be made within the category.

Although fruits are not a free ride in terms of blood sugar and weight, most fruits do contain a variety of vitamins, minerals, and fiber which are important to good health. You'll see from the graphs that some fruits will raise your blood sugar quickly and contribute significantly to weight gain and some will have a small impact on blood sugar and weight gain.

Examples of Fruit Carbohydrates

Many fruits will raise your blood sugar very fast and need to be moderated. The fruits in this category are the following:

pineapples	pears
bananas	grapes
cherries	strawberries
peaches	

Other fruits raise blood sugar less and more slowly and can be eaten more freely. The fruits in this category are the following:

cantaloupe	raspberries
blueberries	grapefruit
blackberries	oranges

I don't mean to imply that fresh fruits are not good for diabetics. But they are not a free ride with regard to blood sugar and weight. Eat more of the fruits on the second list and less of the fruits on the first list.

How About Fruit Juices?

I've found that many fruit juices are problematic because they cause very fast and very big blood sugar increases. In many cases a medium-size glass of *apple* juice or *orange* juice for breakfast will raise my blood sugar more than all the rest of my breakfast combined. And it gets into my bloodstream much faster than I can generally use it so it overworks my pancreas and gets stored in and around my body as fat.

An Associated Press article in the December 11, 2011 edition of the *Honolulu Star* supports what I learned decades ago. The headline states, "Apple juice is far from nutritious, experts say." The article continues "…nutrition experts say apple juice's real danger is to waistlines and children's teeth. Apple juice has few natural nutrients, lots of calories, and in some cases, more sugar than soda. It trains a child to like very sweet things, displaces better beverages and foods, and adds to the obesity problem …".

In my personal experience, apple juice, orange juice, and pine-apple juice all make my blood sugar skyrocket and require me to take far more insulin than the fruits themselves require me to take.

Grapefruit juice does not raise my blood sugar as much or as fast as apple, orange, and pineapple but the increase is still notable. Because of how much these juices impact my blood sugar, I dilute all the juices I drink to about 25 percent juice with about 75 percent water or sparkling mineral water. In other words, one part juice to three parts of water, club soda, or a sparkling water such as Pellegrino or Perrier. You'll soon get used to the less sweet taste in diluted juices.

For anyone trying to lower blood sugar and lose weight, the best juice to drink by far, as you will see in the next chapter, is V-8 juice.

Veggie Carbohydrates

Veggie carbs are more complex than sweet or starchy carbohydrates and you'll see in the graphs they are much slower to enter your bloodstream than either sweet or starchy carbs and slightly slower than most fruit carbs. Most veggie carbohydrates will also raise your blood sugar less than sweet carbs, starchy carbs, or fruit carbs so it gives your overworked pancreas a needed break.

You'll see in the graphs that—except for corn, potatoes, and carrots— the impact of veggie carbs on your blood sugar is neither fast nor significant.

Examples of Veggie Carbohydrates

Because vegetables will cause a very small and very slow increase blood sugar, you will burn most of that small amount of glucose created by veggie carbs before it gets stored around your liver as glycogen or around your body as fat.

These are the foods your mom told you to eat. She was right. They include most vegetables including but not limited to the following:

asparagus	lettuce
broccoli	peppers
tomatoes	mushrooms
cauliflower	peas
brussel sprouts	beans
artichokes	beets
spinach	sauerkraut,
cabbage	salad greens

You can eat as much as you want of these vegetables and—as you will see later—you can use butter freely with them with little or no impact on your blood sugar or weight.

Three vegetables that do cause slightly higher and faster increases than the other vegetables are *corn, potatoes, and carrots.* Although these three foods have much more nutritional benefit than sweet or starchy carbs, you still must moderate your consumption of them and maximize your consumption of the rest of the vegetables.

In the next few chapters you'll see that I speak often of maximizing protein and veggie carbohydrates, moderating fruit carbs, minimizing starchy carbs, and cutting way back on sweet carbohydrates.

Now let's look at protein.

Protein

The molecular structure of protein is more complex than that in the previous four food categories and therefore slower to enter your bloodstream as glucose than sweet carbs, starchy carbs, and fruit carbs, and about as slow as or just slightly slower than most veggie carbs. Just as with veggie carbs, the rise in your blood sugar caused by proteins will be neither fast nor significant.

Protein has gone in and out of favor many times in the past 60 years but from the past 35 years of my blood sugar testing, I've learned that protein has very little effect on my blood sugar and a very noticeably positive effect on my muscle growth when I match protein with moderate strength training.

Because protein will cause neither a quick nor a significant rise in blood sugar, I freely eat large quantities of protein with almost no effect on my blood sugar or weight.

Examples of Protein

Here are examples of protein you can eat often and freely with insignificant impact on blood sugar and weight:

Fish and Seafood

salmon
(wild, not farmed)

halibut

crab

cod

pollock

lobster

trout

shrimp

scallops

Poultry

chicken

turkey

Cornish game hen

(all poultry is okay to eat with the skin but not with breading)

Eggs

Eggs are a mixture of protein and fat that you can eat freely, and will have little impact on your blood sugar, weight, or cholesterol. (More on this later.)

Meat

steak

prime rib

ham

pork chops

bacon

You do *not* have to limit your meats to only lean meat as you will often read. That statement is a holdover from the terribly inaccurate Food Pyramid that triggered the obesity and Type 2 diabetes epidemics. As you study the graphs you'll learn that you can *freely eat* meat marbled with fat and chicken and turkey *with* the skin.

Later in this chapter and in the next two chapters you'll see my defense of fat and read about how medical opinions about fat are quickly evolving.

Although the skin on poultry and the fat on meat is not a problem, *breading* (a starchy carb) on these foods is a problem if you're trying to lower your blood sugars and lose weight.

(As an aside, I personally don't eat veal because of the distressing way calves are confined for their whole lives to improve the taste and tenderness of veal).

My core protein food is Alaskan wild salmon. I eat it two or three times a week in the summer and maybe once or twice a week in the winter.

It's an almost perfect food with very minimal impact on blood sugar. Because it goes in so slowly it gets used before it can be stored as fat on your body. It's very high in protein and high in omega-3 fatty acids, which my secondary research indicates is an exceptionally good fat. Salmon is also a good source of vitamin D. All that and it tastes great too … providing you don't overcook it.

Fats

Not many foods are all or even predominantly fat, but here are a few of the foods that I include in the fat category:

butter	mayonnaise
olive oil	avocados
nuts peanut butter	many salad dressings

Proteins That are High in Fat

These are foods that you can eat freely with little impact on blood sugar and weight—providing you follow my rules on when to eat fat.

eggs (with the yolk)	salmon
pork	most steaks (especially rib eye)
bacon	hamburger
prime rib	bratwurst
spareribs	mutton

Because protein and fat are often present in the same foods, it is difficult to test just fat but more practical to test protein and fat together. Butter and olive oil are exceptions and can be tested with or without protein.

I make a distinction between "natural fats" and processed fats. I'm not personally knowledgeable in the category of processed fats because I don't knowingly eat them and consequently have not tested them. But I am very apprehensive about the taste enhancers and chemicals added during the processing.

Examples of this type of fats I avoid are the following:

margarine	processed sandwich meats
fake butters	precooked frozen lunches and dinners
hot dogs	

Evolving Medical Opinions on Fat

Some doctors and researchers I will refer to later are leading the charge on this issue of fat not being your enemy, but it took over 30 years for the federal bureaucracy to finally—and very quietly—admit the Food Pyramid was wrong and make a change to what they call "My Plate," which is better, but still wrong.

Fats Enter Your Bloodstream Very Slowly

Because the molecular structure of fat is complex and stable, it is slow to break down and enter your bloodstream. That means that you will have more time to burn it as energy before it has a chance to be stored as body fat.

Not only is fat the slowest of the six food groups to enter your bloodstream, but it also has an almost negligible impact on increase in blood sugar. Any impact fat does have on blood sugar is very slow, which means you'll burn it in daily activity before it is stored in your liver as glycogen or around your body as fat.

Let me say this again. *Fat alone has very little impact on your blood sugar or on your weight unless—as you will learn later—it's combined with starchy or sweet carbs.*

Fat Is Your Friend—But a Conditional Friend

I puzzled for years about the fact that proteins with fat for breakfast (bacon and eggs) sometimes raised my blood sugar and insulin demand a lot and sometimes raised it hardly at all. It took me many years of testing my blood to figure out what was happening.

If I didn't eat starchy carbs such as toast, potatoes, or pancakes with my bacon and eggs, that breakfast would have almost no impact on my blood sugar. But if I added toast or potatoes or pancakes or juice to my bacon and eggs, my blood sugar went up more than just the toast, potatoes, pancakes, or juice alone would have caused.

That impact of fats has been the biggest surprise to me over my years of testing. It took me a long time and thousands of blood tests to realize that fat alone has minimal impact on my blood sugar and almost no impact on weight gain. The reason it took me so long is that for years I almost always ate any fatty meats or butter with other foods, often with starchy carbs. Starchy carbs, as you will later see, is bad in combination with fat, especially if eaten in the evening within two hours of going to bed.

My conclusions about fats were confirmed in the tests that I have taken and graphed for this book.

As I said in the lead-in to this section, fat is not the villain it's made out to be. I know this is going to be a hard paradigm shift for Americans, because for years we've read over and over about losing weight with low-fat diets. We've read about low-fat this and low-fat that. Who argued? It seemed so reasonable.

If you don't want to get fat then don't eat fat. It's simple, right?

No ... *wrong.*

Why *Does* Fat Combined with Sweet or Starchy Carbs Impact Your Blood Sugar and Weight Significantly?

The reason those combinations increase blood sugar and weight is very basic. Both sweet carbs and starchy carbs cause fast and big rises in blood sugars. Since foods are all mixed together in the stomach before they are absorbed into the bloodstream, the fat which is usually eaten in smaller quantities than starchy and sweet carbs will be absorbed into the bloodstream along with the high-blood-sugar-creating starchy and sweet carbs.

Fat—although it has more calories per gram than protein or carbs—is normally very slow to enter the bloodstream and is mostly burned or eliminated before it is stored as body fat. But combining fat with sweet or starchy carbs changes all that.

As you'll see in the graphs, a rib-eye steak with vegetables and a salad will have little impact on your blood sugar or weight but combining that rib-eye steak with potatoes or bread allows the nine calories per gram of fat to get into your bloodstream so fast it will be stored in your liver and around your body as body fat before it can be burned.

The same is true for eggs and or bacon for breakfast. The bacon and eggs, alone or in combination, will be very slow to enter your bloodstream and will be burned or eliminated before being stored in your liver or around your body as body fat. If you add toast, pancakes, or even potatoes to the bacon and eggs, your blood sugar will increase dramatically and much of that breakfast will be stored as body fat.

Another combination that causes fat to create high blood sugar and a big weight increase is a meal that includes fat with a sweet dessert. That combination, like the previous example, will result in a much greater weight gain than if the fat and dessert were eaten more than two hours apart.

When you're finished with the next three chapters, I think you'll be convinced that fat alone does not cause high blood sugar nor does it create body fat.

I'll also explain and show evidence of the changing body of research that is showing that fat is not a contributor to bad cholesterol. I'll also demonstrate how nonfat food causes greater increases in blood sugar and weight than the same food and brand with fat.

Finally, I'll show you which health and fitness organizations have eliminated restrictions on dietary fat.

I know this is counter to everything we've all been told for so many years. It also seems counter to what sounds like straightforward logic: If you put fat in your mouth it must somehow transform into body fat and make its way to your waist or hips or your butt. It's been an easy sell for the Government when it said, "If you don't want to get fat don't eat fat." An easy sell *but wrong*!

If you are one of those few Americans who want to gain weight, don't bother trying to do it by eating a lot of natural fats because it's not going to happen. In the words of Dr. Rob Benedetti, the chair of the Medical Division of Rockwood Clinic in Spokane, "Nobody ever got fat by eating too many avocados."

If you *do* want to gain weight your best strategy is to follow the Food Pyramid that for many decades guided America's dietary habits.

What do Others Say About the Role of Fat in a Healthy Diet?

In the next chapters, I'll be explaining how the results of my tests and experiences measuring my own blood sugar are gaining support in the research and medical communities. I'll also be referring you to medical researchers and doctors who argue convincingly that it's not fat that creates high cholesterol and high triglycerides levels, which are the big precursors of circulatory and heart problems. It's sweet carbs and starchy carbs that cause those problems.

Now let's look at the graphs that can change your life.

Chapter 5

Graphics of Good Foods and Bad Foods for Type 2 Diabetics

Testing Food Impact on Blood Sugar—
60,000 Tests and Counting
It's taken me 35 years, and over 60,000 blood sugar tests, to learn what you will learn in these next three chapters about food.

Before Self-testing
Though I'm in my 54th year and counting with Type 1 diabetes, self-testing has been available for only about 38 years. In the years before self-testing the only way I could get a blood sugar measurement was to set an appointment with my doctor, who would give me a lab request. I then had to go to a lab to have a blood sample taken from a vein in my arm. The local lab sent it out to an analytical lab and got the result back in three days. The local lab would then call my doctor, who had a staff person call me and tell me what my blood sugar had been three or four days prior. Because of that cumbersome process, I had my blood sugar tested only three or four times a year during my first 16 or so years with diabetes.

After Self-testing

Now I self-test when I wake up each morning, before and after most meals, often between meals, and twice before I go to bed each night—about an hour apart. I also test before physical activities and any other time I think my blood sugar needs adjusting. As a result of all these tests I've learned how hundreds—perhaps thousands—of different foods and combinations of foods impact my blood sugar and weight. I've learned not only how *much* but also how *fast* different foods raise my blood sugar.

What I Can't Measure

This is a good time to state that I can't make any judgments from my empirical testing of foods regarding their content of vitamins, minerals, or other ingredients that don't relate to blood sugar.

What I Can Measure

What I can and do measure, of course, is blood sugar and that is a huge factor in your general health. High blood sugars, over time negatively affect your pancreas, your kidneys, your liver, your heart, your feet, and your vision.

Improving your blood sugar control will dramatically improve your health and your life expectancy.

Who Will Benefit from This Information

This information is written primarily for people with pre-diabetes, borderline diabetes, or Type 2 diabetes. However, it also applies directly to the two thirds of American adults who the Center for Disease Control says are overweight or obese and would like to lose weight. And it will be beneficial to all those who would just like to live a longer, healthier life.

The Purpose of the Graphs

The purpose of the graphs I present in this chapter is to provide visual representations of what I've learned from the 60,000 blood tests I have given myself over the past 35 years. These graphs will make it easier for the readers to visualize and remember which food groups—and foods within the groups—elevate blood sugars and add weight and which food groups and foods do not.

As you now know, since I'm a Type 1 diabetic, my body produces no insulin at all but whatever foods or combinations of foods I eat are converted to glucose in my blood just as they are for everyone, diabetic or not. But if I don't give myself a shot of insulin when I eat that food, my blood sugar will just keep on rising until I do give myself a shot.

Eating foods and not giving myself any insulin for 90 minutes is precisely how I can measure the blood sugar impact and therefore fat-gain impact of individual foods and combinations of foods.

The graphs are a result of very specific tests on blood sugar impact and therefore weight gain impact of multiple foods and combinations of foods in the six food groups.

Remember, I break down foods into the following six groups based on their impact on blood sugar and weight. You'll recall those six groups are:

sweet carbs	veggie carbs
starchy carbs	protein
fruit carbs	fat

The graphs will clearly show what foods you should minimize to avoid large increases in blood sugar and therefore weight gain and what foods you can *maximize* with little rise in blood sugar and therefore weight loss. The results will surprise you ... and change your life.

My Methodology for Testing

Over the past 35 years of eating and testing my blood sugar and trying to match my insulin injections to foods I've eaten, I've learned a lot about which foods cause the greatest blood sugar increases and weight gain and which cause the least blood sugar increases and weight gain. I've continually adjusted my selection of foods to respond to that information.

But for the purposes of developing the graphs in this book I've conducted tests with a very specific and consistent protocol.

I first made sure my blood sugar was stable. To assure stability, most of my tests were done in the morning when I hadn't eaten anything for at least 10 hours. To confirm that my blood sugar was stable, I tested two or three times before I ate or drank the foods or drinks to be tested.

Once I was sure my blood sugar was stable, I consumed the test foods or drinks. The next step was to set my smart phone to alert me every 10 minutes for 90 minutes.

I made a special effort to keep my activity constant during the tests so the results wouldn't be skewed even slightly by more or less activity. I usually read the paper, a magazine, or a book during the tests. During those tests I was nine steps away from the counter upon which my testers and the charts were placed. That meant 18 steps back and forth every 10 minutes for each test. Counting duplicate tests to confirm results, on average I stuck my fingers and tested about 12 to 15 times within every 90-minute period.

At the end of 90 minutes and after all the results were recorded, I took an appropriate shot of insulin which—in a little more than an hour—brought my blood sugar back to a normal range.

Those 90 minutes tell a dramatic, visual story. They tell a story that can improve the lives of millions of Americans; a story that can help millions of Type 2 diabetics lower their blood sugars, reverse their diabetes, and lose weight. It will also prevent millions of Americans from ever getting Type 2 diabetes in the first place.

Indexing the Tests

The final point I need to make in describing my methodology is that at whatever stable point my blood was when I started, I indexed it to 100. What that means is if I established that my starting blood sugar was say 112 and stable, then my index was minus 12. That means I subtracted 12 points from my starting level and 12 points from every measurement for the full 90 minutes. And if for example my starting point was 84, I added 16 points to my starting level and 16 to each test for the full 90 minutes. That process gives every test the same starting point and will show accurate slopes, peaks, and areas that can be easily compared.

The findings are dramatic and likely different from what you've read or been told about food. The conclusions will change your eating lifestyle, your health and your enjoyment of life. It's not about a short-term diet but rather about eating in a healthy way that you will enjoy for the rest of your life—eating *smaller* portions of the foods that maximize your blood sugars and contribute to weight gain, and eating *larger* portions of the foods that have minimal effect on blood sugars and which will contribute to weight loss.

Will the Foods I've Graphed Have the Same Impact on Everyone Else as They Have Had on Me?

The answer is, in general, yes. In terms of speed of entry into the bloodstream and impacts on blood sugar and weight, foods act the same for everyone.

There is, however, a variation of impact based on size. People of different size have different volumes of blood circulating through their bodies, so the impact will vary based on the volume of blood. A small female may have as little as five pints of blood circulating through her body but a large male could have 10 pints or more circulating in his body.

If a very small female, for example, ate the same size portions of foods I did, the impact on her blood sugar and weight would be proportionally greater than the impact on my blood sugar. If a 260-pound male (I weigh 190) ate the same foods and portion sizes I did, the impact on his blood sugar would be proportionally less than the impact on my blood sugar and weight.

It's the same as putting a teaspoon of sugar in an 8-ounce glass of iced tea compared to putting a teaspoon of sugar in a 16-ounce glass of iced tea. The 8-ounce glass of iced tea would be twice as sweet.

Although the numbers shown on my tests would not be precisely the same for everyone, the slopes, the peaks, and the shaded area of the graphs will still give a valid comparison of foods to each other. For example, if food "A" causes my blood sugar to rise *faster and more* than food "B", it would do the same for you. If food "C" causes my blood sugar to *rise more slowly and less* than food "D" it will do the same for you.

Not Just Memorizing What to Eat but Understanding Why

From 1985 through 1989, I chaired the US Olympic Committee's bids for the Olympic Winter Games. During those years, Anchorage was America's candidate.

I spoke around the world promoting Anchorage as a host city for the Winter Olympics. Our committee also hosted a number of International Olympic Committee (IOC) members on visits to Anchorage.

One of the visitors we hosted was the IOC member from China. After his visit to Anchorage he made a comment to me that I have never forgotten. As we were riding together to the airport for his return trip home he turned to me and said, "Mr. Chairman, I've heard you speak at many meetings around the world but I've forgotten much of what you said about Anchorage being an ideal host for the

Olympic Winter Games. But when I saw your visual presentations, I remembered. Now that I've visited your city, I understand."

I think the visual presentations of the graphs will help you remember. But when you start seeing the resulting improved blood sugars and weight loss, *you'll understand.*

Using the Graphs

The graphs you are about to review have five major elements that you need to understand.

The horizontal axis of the graphs is the line across the bottom of the graph. It's labeled 0 through 90 minutes and represents the time in minutes that I measured the change in my blood sugars.

The vertical axis of the graphs is the line along the left side of the graph and it represents the rise in blood sugar measured in milligrams per deciliter (mg/dl). Note that it starts at 100—a very normal number—not at zero.

The slope of the graphs is the angled line and represents speed of the rise in blood sugar.

The *steeper the slope*, the faster the rise in blood sugar (glucose). Remember, a fast rise in blood sugar usually means the glucose will be stored as a form of fat before you get a chance to burn it. That's bad.

The *flatter the slope*, the slower the rise in blood sugar. A slow rise usually means much of the glucose will be burned before it ever gets stored as fat. That's good.

The peak of the graphs shows how hard your pancreas is asked to work to get that food out of the bloodstream and into the cells. This is very important for pre-diabetics, borderline diabetics, and Type 2 diabetics who wish to reverse their diabetes. It is so important it warrants a repeat, in different words, of something I said in chapter 1.

If you're a Type 2 diabetic, borderline diabetic, or pre-diabetic, it's likely that less-than-healthy eating habits and maybe a sedentary life style over a number of years or decades have been causing your pancreas to work overly hard to get glucose (sugar) from your bloodstream into your cells.

Those bad habits may not have shown up as high blood sugar for decades because your pancreas compensated by producing more insulin. But now your pancreas is, in effect, overworked and tired, and not producing enough insulin to get all the excess glucose out of your bloodstream into the cells. Hence, you have higher-than-normal blood sugars and now have or will have Type 2 diabetes.

The fact that your pancreas has likely been overworked illustrates how important the peak of the graphs is. The peak reflects how hard your pancreas will work to get that glucose out of the bloodstream into your cells. In other words, if a food or combination of foods raises your blood sugar by 200 mg/dl your pancreas will work twice as hard as it would if a food or combination of foods raises your blood sugar by only 100 mg/dl.

At either the pre-diabetic, borderline diabetic, or Type 2 diabetic stage, you will not likely ever see your blood sugars as high as mine are for the tests. The reason is that your pancreas is producing *some* insulin which has a lowering effect on your blood sugar.

So even though you won't see blood sugars as high as the peaks of the graphs show, they do tell you how hard that food is making your pancreas work.

You must do everything you can to lighten the workload of your pancreas. So please pay attention to the *peaks* of the graphs.

The shaded area of the graphs *represents the comparative weight gain that food or combination of foods will have.* The faster the food causes your blood sugar to rise and the greater the rise, the more weight you will gain as illustrated by the gray area of the graphs.

The foods or combination of foods that cause your blood sugar to rise less and to rise more slowly will result in weight loss. This is a crucial statement. Please read it again and lock it into your mind.

Much like the pancreas's work is represented by the *peak* of the graphs, the shaded area is not intended to represent a specific weight gain of ounces or grams but rather a comparison of one food to another. For example, since the *shaded area* of graph 1 is roughly five times as large as a shaded area of graph 42, the contribution to weight of the food in graph 1 will be five times as great as the contribution to weight in graph 42.

My Daily Feedback on the Impact of Foods on Weight

Non-Type 1 diabetics can get feedback on the impact of foods on weight only *once or twice a week or once or twice a month* when they step on a scale. They can only speculate as to which of the foods they ate contributed to weight gain or loss. I get feedback on individual foods between six and ten times a day and a summary result at the end of each day.

This information is so valuable it can positively impact the lives of millions of people. I hope you are one of them.

Why Counting Calories Doesn't Work Very Well

Although authors continually promote counting calories, Americans keep getting fatter and fatter. What's the reason? The reason is, not all calories are the same. As you review the graphs you'll see that 200 calories of protein, vegetables, and—yes—even fat will raise your blood sugar a lot less and contribute less to your weight gain than 200 calories of sweet or starchy carbs.

To illustrate, compare a 214-calorie Hershey bar (graph 4) to three eggs cooked different ways (graphs 42, 43, and 44), about 213 calories. Because a Hershey bar gets into your bloodstream much faster and ends with a much higher blood sugar, the gray area is about six times greater than the gray area of three eggs. That means a Hershey bar will cause weight gain approximately six times more than three eggs and will make your pancreas work much harder.

As you study the graphs you'll see over and over that it's not the calories but the category of food that counts.

One well-respected researcher and author, Gary Taubes, who wrote *Good Calories, Bad Calories*, explains convincingly that "obesity is caused, not by the quantity of calories you eat but by the quality. Carbohydrates, particularly refined ones like white bread and pasta, raise insulin levels, promoting the storage of fat."

The results of my study show that all starchy carbs and sweet carbs raise insulin levels significantly—as shown by the shaded area of the graphs—and promote the storage of fat.

The only time you should pay attention to calories is when you're comparing foods in the same category. If you're comparing *starchy carbs to starchy carbs, sweet carbs to sweet carbs*, looking at calories has some meaning.

The Value of Having Six Food Groups Instead of Just Three

As you review the graphs, it's most important that you go back and forth to understand how the six different groups compare with one another.

No one can tell you how much *every* food you'll ever eat will contribute to your blood sugar and weight. Even if they could, no one could memorize all that and use it in a functional way.

Your primary goal should be to understand which food *groups* are the biggest contributors to high blood sugar and weight gain and which are not.

Applying the Graphs

Now let's look at how different foods impact blood sugar and weight. By the time you finish reviewing these graphs you'll have a strong visual memory of which foods you must *minimize* to lower blood sugar and lose weight and which foods you can *maximize* with little or no impact on weight gain.

Once the graphs have found a secure place in your memory they will always be there. You'll always remember which food groups and which foods within those groups contribute more to blood sugar and weight gain and which will contribute less to blood sugar and will result in weight loss.

By understanding and applying the information in these graphs, Type 2 diabetics will lower their blood sugars, lose weight, and avoid devastating complications associated with diabetes. Pre-diabetics or borderline diabetics will avoid ever getting Type 2 diabetes in the first place.

Some Notes on the Graphs

As you review these graphs, you'll see that foods typical to breakfasts are measured and graphed more often than other meals.

There are two reasons I've done this. First, people tend to eat the same or similar foods most mornings for breakfast, so getting into a better pattern of eating is easier. Second, there seems to be more misinformation about healthy breakfast foods than about other meals. But because I've been testing for so long and so frequently, I know that whatever the meal, breakfast, lunch, dinner, or snacks, all the foods within the six food groups act similarly.

The final note before you get into the graphs is that you will see some graphs have slight dips between 40 and 70 minutes. This happens because my pump is putting a tiny maintenance amount of insulin into my body continuously. It's called the basal rate. Not unlike the small amount of glycogen put into the body by the liver.

What that small decrease reflects is my body using a small amount of that glucose just walking up to my tester and back to my seat. My body would use roughly the same amount for all foods tested but in some cases glucose is going in so fast that a slight dip doesn't show. This effect does not significantly change the results.

Sweet Carbohydrates

I'm going to start with sweet carbs. We all know they make your blood sugar go up and contribute substantially to weight gain. No surprise there. But these graphs will give readers perspective on how much and how fast this happens. It also gives a point of reference for the rest of the food categories.

Here's a review of foods in this category:

Sweetened (non-diet) soft drinks, candy bars, cakes, pies, donuts, sweet rolls, sweet toppings for ice creams, chocolates, caramels, other sweetened candies, sweet desserts. We all know by now that too much sugar is a villain. Then what about all the *sugar-free* candies? Are they okay? They taste just like regular candy. But look closely at the label. You'll see that many of those items are sweetened with high-fructose corn syrup or with other sweeteners like sucrose— not much different than cane sugars but a little more concentrated ... and therefore worse for you.

Don't think you're doing yourself a favor by eating *sugar-free* candy. It only means the manufacturers have likely used concentrated sweeteners other than sugar. Both regular candy and sugar-free candy are items that you need to start minimizing or better yet, eliminating. This is, of course, not new information but if you do all the other things I'll propose and still eat lots of sweets, you're not going to make the progress you need or want.

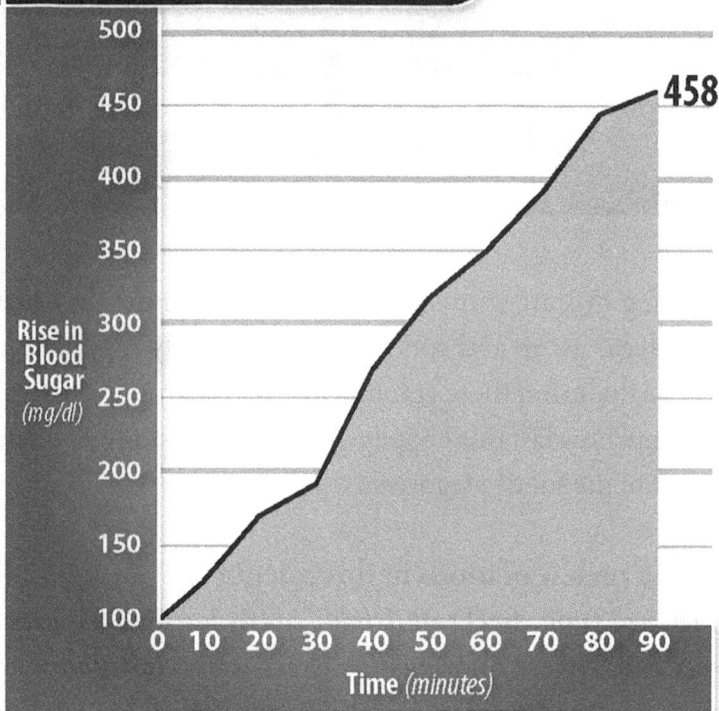

1 **Cherry danish sweet roll**

Total Calories – 440

Cherry Danish

This is my record holder for increasing my blood sugar. It went from 100 to 458 mg/dl in 90 minutes. This caused a net blood sugar rise* of 358 mg/dl in 90 minutes. As you'll see when you review other graphs, this is a huge rise and a great contributor to weight.

---

* Notice that the net blood sugar rise is 100 points less than my final blood sugar on the graph. The reason is, of course, that all my blood sugars start or are indexed to 100, which is within the generally accepted normal.

2 | **One slice apple pie**

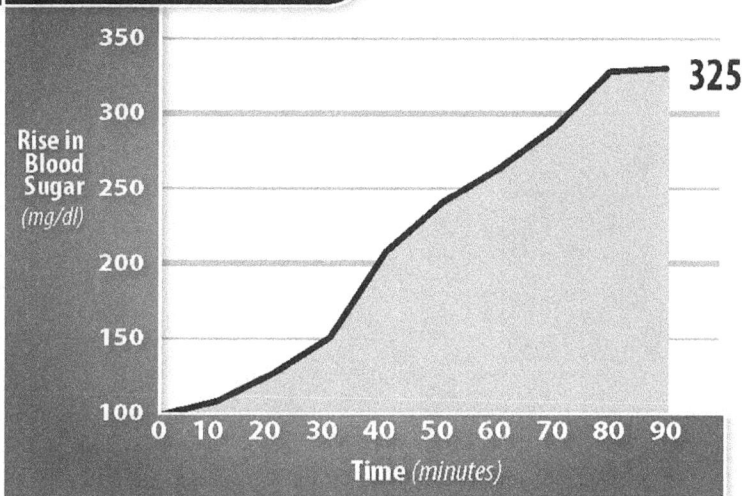

Rise in Blood Sugar (mg/dl)

350
300
250
200
150
100

325

0 10 20 30 40 50 60 70 80 90

Time *(minutes)*

Total Calories – 277

Apple Pie

This is another very big rise in blood sugar. In my experience this blood sugar rise is typical of most pies. Whether you cut out desserts like this, eat them much less frequently, or dramatically reduce portion size will be up to you. The important thing right now is to lock this visual in your mind. Most pies and cakes will act similarly to this. Though I eat pie or cake only about three or four times a year, their combination of sweet carbs and starchy carbs have always caused the biggest rises in my blood sugars. I can cover it with a huge infusion of insulin that is often larger than the infusion for the complete meal preceding it. That means the pie or cake would raise my blood sugar more and make me fatter than all the rest of the food on my plate combined.

| 3 | Chocolate covered donut |

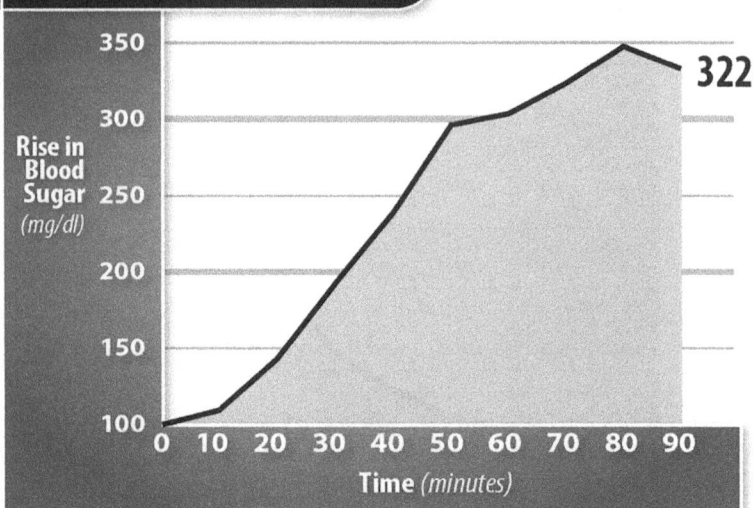

Rise in Blood Sugar (mg/dl)

322

Time (minutes)

Total Calories – 276

Chocolate-Covered Donut

Here's another food that has an impact even greater than most would expect. Donuts are a very common breakfast habit for many people. If you eat a donut or a sweet roll for breakfast and wonder why you're gaining weight, compare this graph to other breakfast choices shown in later graphs.

4 — Hershey Bar

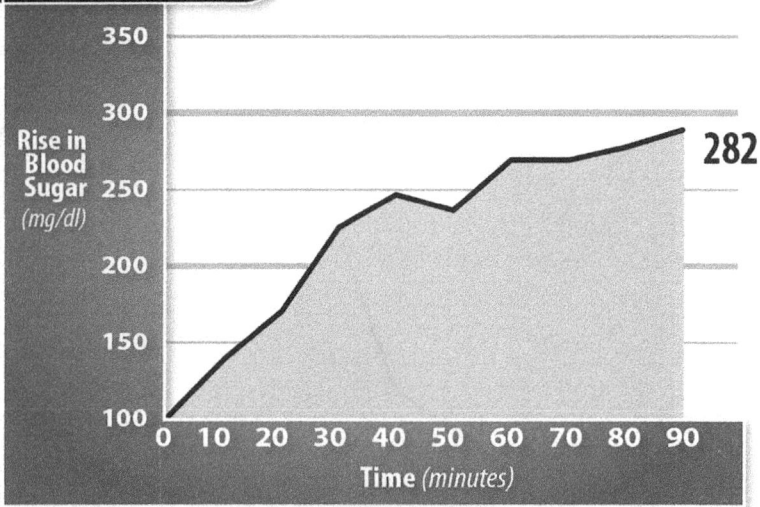

Rise in Blood Sugar *(mg/dl)*

350
300
250
200
150
100

282

0 10 20 30 40 50 60 70 80 90

Time *(minutes)*

Total Calories – 214

Hershey Bar

I've included a Hershey bar graph because it is such a common candy bar and people can relate to it. Both the slope and the impact are less than the first three graphs but still significant. A Hershey bar has 214 calories. Compare this graph to eggs (graphs 42, 43, and 44). Three large eggs have 210 to 214 calories total but have about one fifth the impact on blood sugar and weight that a Hershey bar does. Remember calories are pertinent only if one is comparing foods from the same group.

5 | ***Coke*** One 16.9 fl oz Bottle

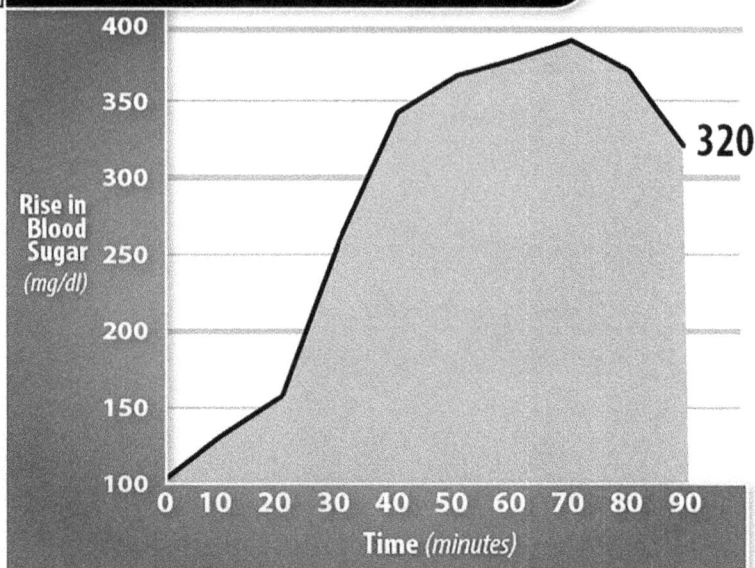

400

350

300

Rise in
Blood
Sugar 250
(mg/dl)

200

150

100

0 10 20 30 40 50 60 70 80 90

320

Time *(minutes)*

Total Calories – 200

Coke

I've included a graph of a 500 ml bottle of Coca Cola which is the most common size I've found in stores. It gets into your bloodstream very quickly, which is bad because you will not likely burn that glucose before it is stored in your liver as glycogen and around your body as body fat.

6 | **Haagen Dazs Zesty Lemon Sorbet**

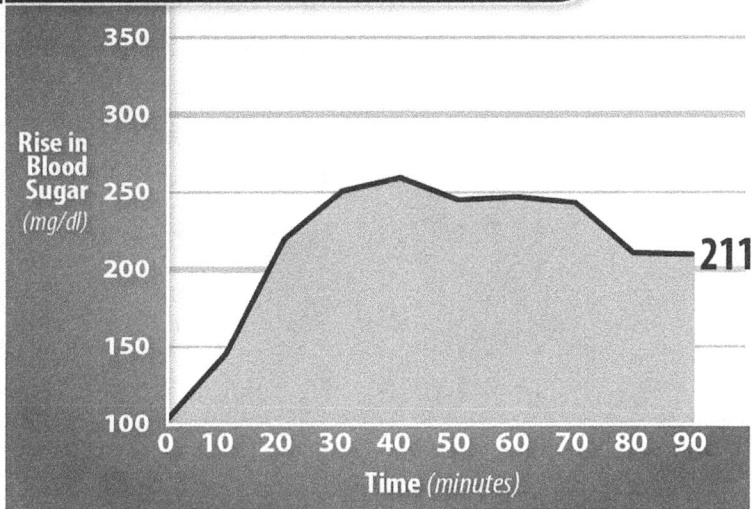

Total Calories – 120

Ice Cream or Sorbet

I'm sorry to report that ice cream in its various forms is a big contributor to blood sugar elevation and weight gain. The combination of sweet carbs and fat is not good. You'll learn later in this book why you should avoid eating ice cream late in the evening. If you really love ice cream—doesn't everyone—and can't do without it, eat it earlier in the day and do everything you can to minimize it. For a smaller impact—as well as a great taste, I periodically eat Haagen Daz Zesty Lemon Sorbet.

For this test, I ate about one half of a half-pint container, which is a lot for me. When I do eat it, I typically eat just a couple of tablespoons at a time so a pint may last me a month. But it is very refreshing.

Conclusions Regarding the Sweet Carbohydrates Group

We all know sweets are contributors to high blood sugars and weight gain. But after you review all the graphs you'll see just how significant the blood sugar increases and weight gains are.

You can eat three eggs for breakfast for a week and gain less weight that having one sugared soft drink or one sweet roll. In addition, eating three eggs for breakfast for a week puts a lot less strain on an overworked pancreas.

Starchy Carbohydrates

My next category of foods based on the speed of absorption and total impact on blood sugar and weight is starchy carbohydrates. As a reminder, here are some examples of foods I include in this category: *waffles, pancakes, breakfast cereals, white breads, multigrain breads, (Whole-grain bread is better than multigrain), rolls, bagels, buns, muffins, tortillas, tortilla chips, potato chips, spaghetti, lasagna, pasta, white rice, crackers, and wheat products in general.*

I also categorize *corn* and *potatoes* as starchy carbohydrates because of the speed and amount of blood sugar increase they cause. In other words, even though they are considered vegetables, they act like starchy carbs in terms of blood sugar increases and weight gain.

| 7 | Spaghetti without butter or sauce |

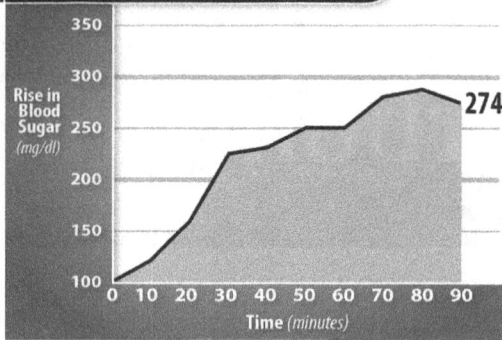

Rise in Blood Sugar (mg/dl)

274

Time (minutes)

Total Calories – 220

| 8 | Spaghetti w/ Butter |

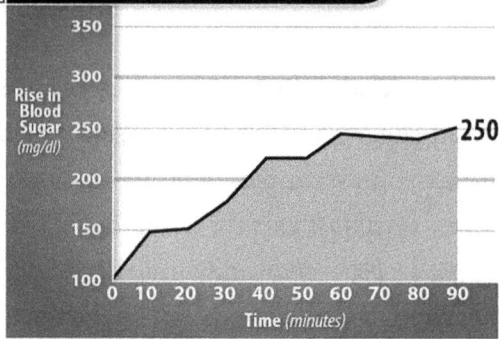

Rise in Blood Sugar (mg/dl)

250

Time (minutes)

Total Calories – 310

Spaghetti

This graph shows the impact of a starchy carbohydrate if eaten without sauce, butter, or other flavorings. Normally it would not be eaten this way but my purpose in this graph is to illustrate the blood sugar and weight gain impact of just starchy carbs. Note how much more slowly blood sugar goes up when fat (butter) is added to the spaghetti. If I had tested for more than 90 minutes you would see that the spaghetti with butter would continue to raise blood sugar longer than spaghetti without butter. But this slower, longer rise gives you more time to burn the glucose before it is stored.

9 | **1/2 Plain Baked Potato**

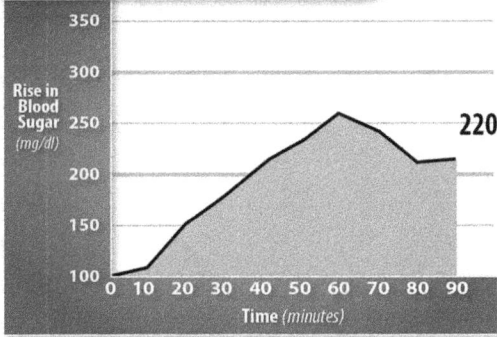

220

Total Calories – 100

10 | **1/2 Baked Potato w/ Butter&SourCrm.**

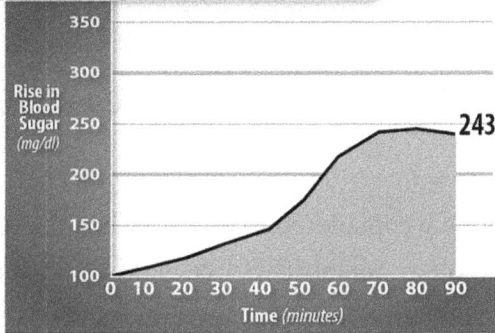

243

Total Calories – 235

Potatoes

Note how much more slowly potatoes with butter and sour cream enter the bloodstream. This gives you a better chance to burn the glucose before it gets stored. We would all be better off if we ate half as much potato with twice as much butter and sour cream. You'll see what I mean when I get to the "fat" graphs.

11 — One Minute Quaker Oats oatmeal w/ fat free milk
(No sugar added)

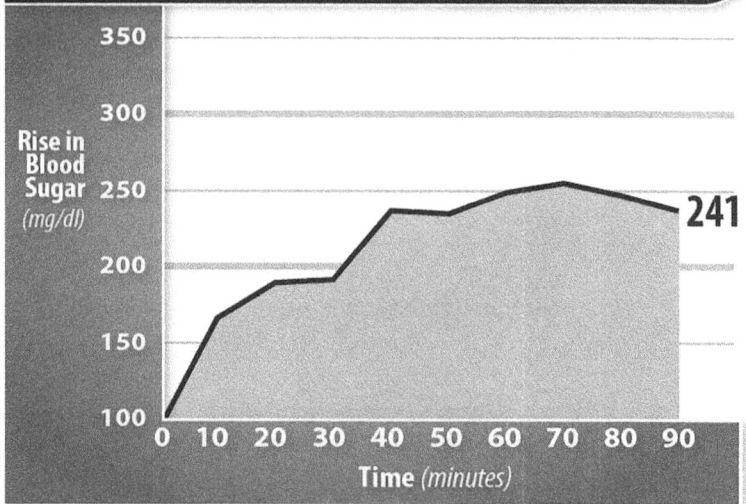

Rise in Blood Sugar *(mg/dl)*

350
300
250 — **241**
200
150
100

Time *(minutes)*: 0 10 20 30 40 50 60 70 80 90

Total Calories – 230

Oatmeal

Oatmeal is widely considered to be a very healthy breakfast but it is similar to the other cereals that I've graphed with regard to blood sugar and weight contribution. However, as you continue with this chapter, you will see that other choices will be better for blood sugar control and weight loss. I'm not recommending that you not eat oatmeal only that you need to be careful. It's not a free ride.

12 | 1 Cup *Special K* w/ Fat Free Milk
(No sugar added)

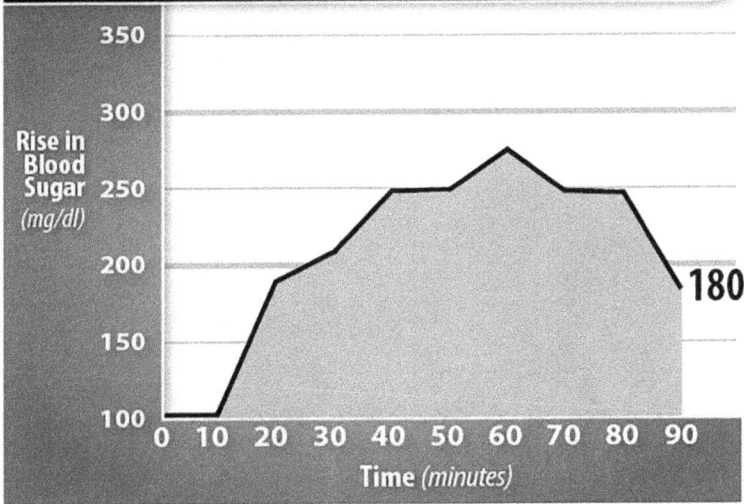

Rise in Blood Sugar *(mg/dl)*

350
300
250
200
150
100

Time *(minutes)*: 0 10 20 30 40 50 60 70 80 90

180

Total Calories – 200

Cereal

Most cereals seem to identify about the same range of calories in their nutrition facts—usually between 100 and 130 but as you will see later, calories and blood sugar, and calories and weight gain are not always related. Some foods with fewer calories may have more impact on blood sugar and weight gain than other foods with more calories. When you compare these cereal graphs with graphs of two eggs, which have about the same number of calories, you'll begin to understand that statement.

I don't eat much cereal because of the big impact on my blood sugar and weight but I chose Total and Special K to test because it looked the healthiest from the box information. The results of these tests are quite consistent with my general experience with many different cereals. Of the cereals that I have eaten, General Mills' Fiber One has the least impact on my blood sugar and therefore on weight gain, but even with that cereal you need to keep the portion size small.

13 | One cup *Cheerios* with fat free milk, no sugar

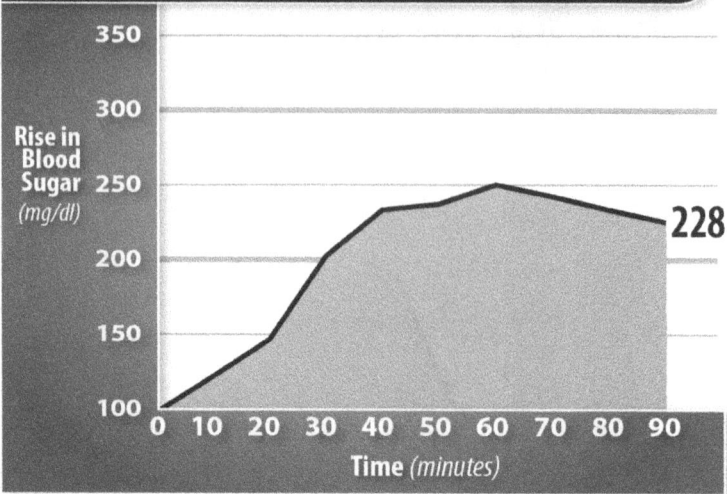

Rise in Blood Sugar *(mg/dl)*

350
300
250
200
150
100

0 10 20 30 40 50 60 70 80 90

228

Time *(minutes)*

Net blood sugar rise – 128

14 | One cup *Total* with fat free milk, 1 tsp sugar

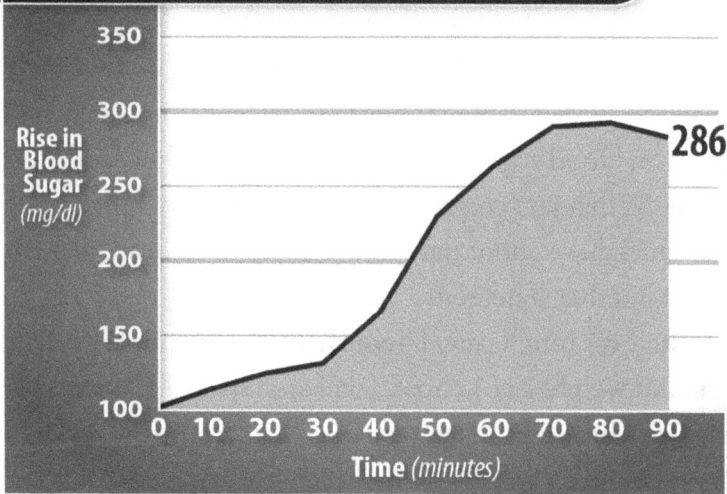

Rise in Blood Sugar *(mg/dl)*

350
300
250
200
150
100

0 10 20 30 40 50 60 70 80 90

286

Time *(minutes)*

Net blood sugar rise – 186

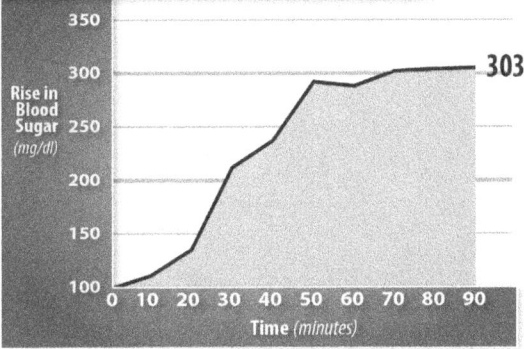

15 One cup Total and whole milk *(No sugar added)*

Net blood sugar rise – 203

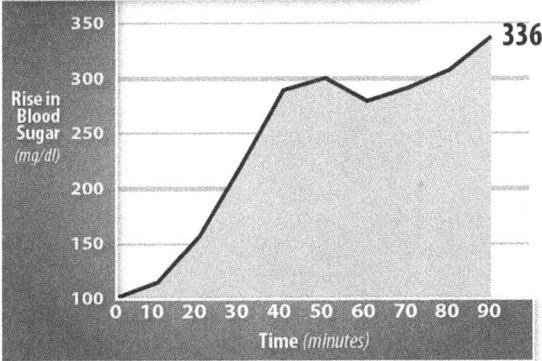

16 Granola and fat free milk *(No sugar added)*

Total Calories – 406

Granola

I don't recall ever eating granola as a breakfast cereal before this test so I didn't know what to expect. But, like many Americans, I always associated granola with good health so I was very surprised by the results of my testing.

Granola is popular among runners and for good reason. A small bowl of granola is ideal for giving your body a large influx of glucose. Perfect if you're going on a five-mile training run after eating but not good if you're going to the office or relaxing after eating it.

17 — 1/2 Bagel with cream cheese

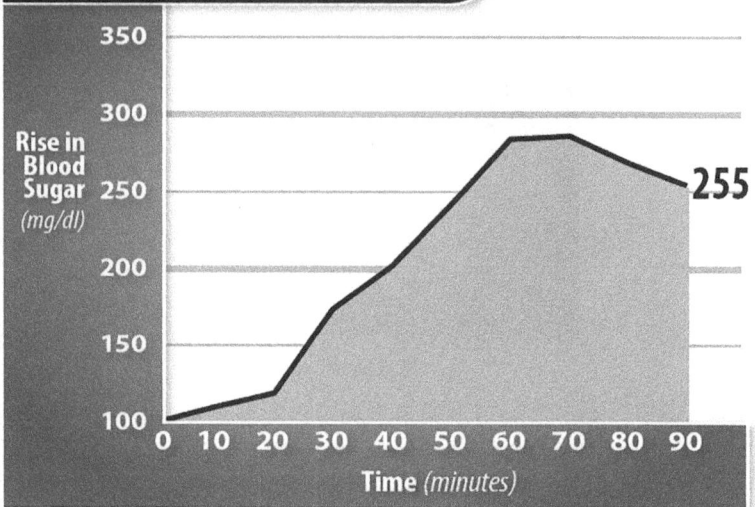

Rise in Blood Sugar (mg/dl)

255

Time (minutes)

Total Calories – 219

Bagels

Bagels seem to be a food that people who are health conscious eat. I've often heard folks say with a certain modicum of self-pride, "I usually just have a bagel and cream cheese for breakfast." With that statement in mind, I tested, not a full bagel, but one half bagel with cream cheese and then a bagel without cream cheese or butter. If this is what a half bagel does, think about the impact of a full bagel. You'd be getting into Cherry Danish territory.

18 | 1/2 Bagel w/ vs w/o Butter

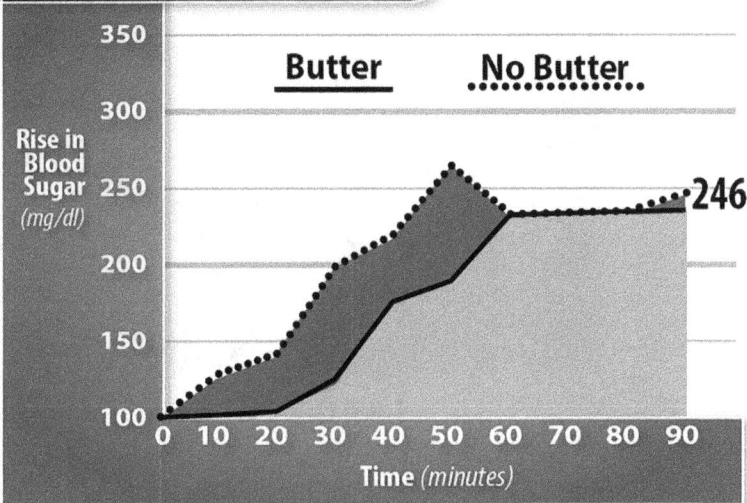

Butter ......**No Butter**......

Rise in
Blood
Sugar
(mg/dl)

350
300
250 ....**246**
200
150
100

0 10 20 30 40 50 60 70 80 90

Time (minutes)

Total Calories – 260w/Butter | 160w/o

On graph 18, the light gray area is a bagel with butter. The dark gray added to the light gray is a bagel without butter. The butter slows down the entry of glucose into the bloodstream and gives you more opportunity to burn the glucose before it gets stored.

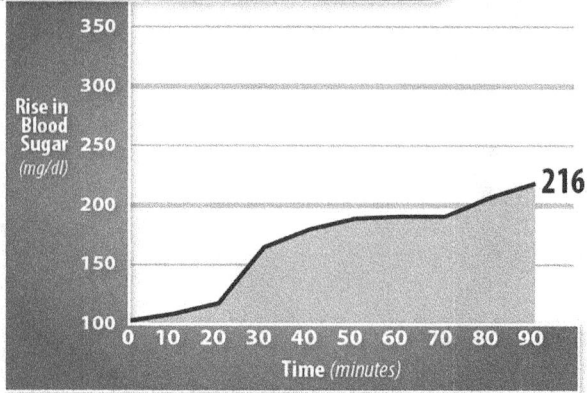

19 | **One slice wheat toast without butter**

216

Total Calories – 69

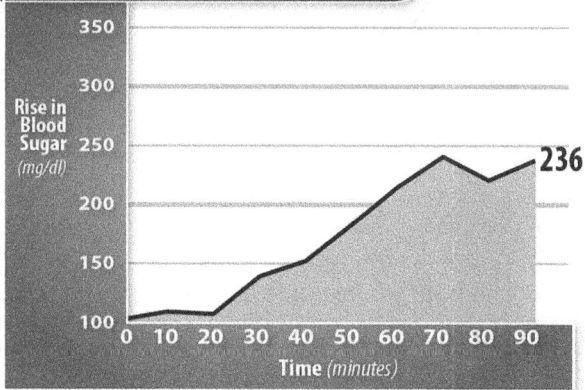

20 | **One slice wheat toast with butter**

236

Total Calories – 90

Wheat Toast

When I do eat toast, which is not often anymore, I choose whole-wheat toast. From everything I've read, whole-wheat toast is better than white toast. I can't measure that, but as I have with cereal, I've gradually reduced the number of bread products I eat because of their discouragingly high increases in my blood sugar and therefore weight from them.

21 | **Gluten free toast with butter**

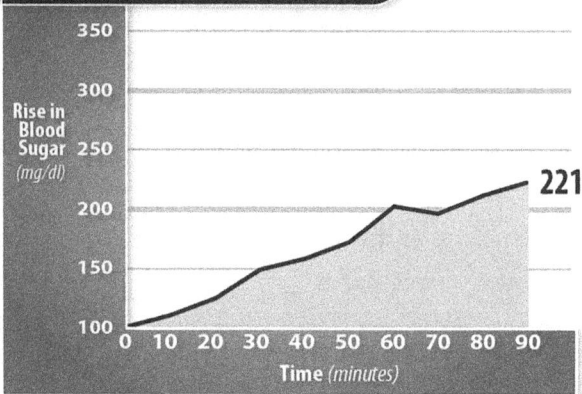

Rise in Blood Sugar (mg/dl)

221

Time (minutes)

Total Calories – 91

Gluten-Free Toast

Gluten-free toast is not something I'm familiar with nor have I eaten it prior to the tests graphed below so I can't say that the few tests I took are absolute certainties, but the cornstarch and tapioca starch in gluten-free bread appear to have a slightly smaller impact on my blood sugar than the wheat in other breads.

Conclusions on Starchy Carbohydrates

It's been my experience as a result of thousands of blood sugar tests that starchy carbs raise my blood sugar almost as much as sweet carbs. I'm not suggesting that sweet carbs and starchy carbs are equivalent in terms of general health. I'm confident that starchy carbs are the better, but if you want to lower blood sugars, control blood sugar swings, and lose weight, dramatically reducing starchy carbs is absolutely necessary.

A Note on Healthy, Active Children

This is a good point to remind readers that the eating suggestions I make here are geared toward adults and not young, active, growing children. If children are overweight or obese they would do well by following the advice in my eating recommendations, but if they're of normal weight, active, and growing these recommendations are not for them— especially with regard to starchy carbs. Children who are going out to play for three or four hours after breakfast will do fine with cereal and toast but if they're going to sit in a classroom or in front of a computer or television they should cut back somewhat on starchy carbs for breakfast.

Once you see the graphs of how the next four categories of foods act you'll begin to be able to visually compare how much starchy carbs and sweet carbs contribute to high blood sugar and weight gain.

Fruit Carbohydrates

The foods in this category are quite obvious. Almost everyone knows what fruits are: *apples, oranges, pineapples, bananas, watermelons, peaches, pears, berries, and so forth.*

Fruit carbs are certainly better than sweet carbs and starchy carbs in terms of blood sugar and weight control. They also are known to provide more healthful nutrients than the first two categories. But are they a free ride? Can you eat as much fruit as you wish without significant blood sugar increases and weight gain? I'll start with the fruits that have the highest impact on blood sugar and weight gain and move to fruits with lower impact on blood sugar and weight.

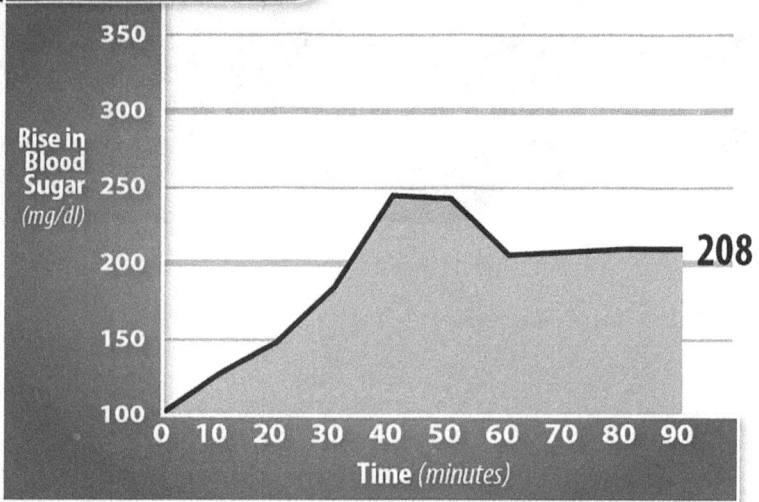

22 | One large banana

Rise in Blood Sugar (mg/dl)

350
300
250
200
150
100

208

0 10 20 30 40 50 60 70 80 90

Time (minutes)

Total Calories – 121

Bananas

Bananas have the highest impact on my blood sugar of the common fruits I eat. I stopped eating pineapples because they raised my blood sugar so much. That, I think, is obvious to most people because of the extraordinary sweetness of that fruit. But bananas don't have that sweet taste so their impact would be hard for someone to tell just based on taste. In the graph, you'll see that the impact of a banana on blood sugar and its contribution to weight gain are big. You'll also notice a drop at about 50 minutes which I explained just prior to the graph section. Consider for a moment adding a banana to the cereal graphs you just saw. That combination creates a big, big impact on blood sugar and a substantial contribution to weight gain.

23 **One cup Queen Anne cherries**

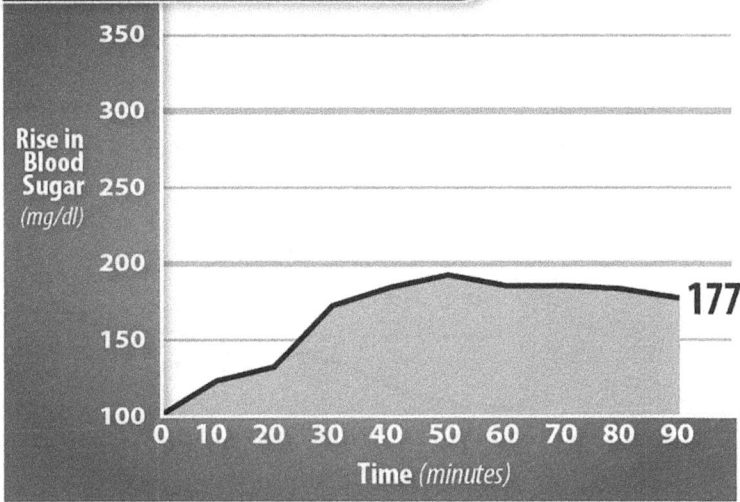

Rise in Blood Sugar *(mg/dl)*

350
300
250
200
150
100

177

0 10 20 30 40 50 60 70 80 90

Time *(minutes)*

Total Calories – 91

Queen Anne Cherries

I eat a small to moderate number of cherries—usually Queen Anne or Bing cherries. Cherries have only a moderate impact on blood sugar. They're a good snack but don't overindulge.

24 | **One large orange**

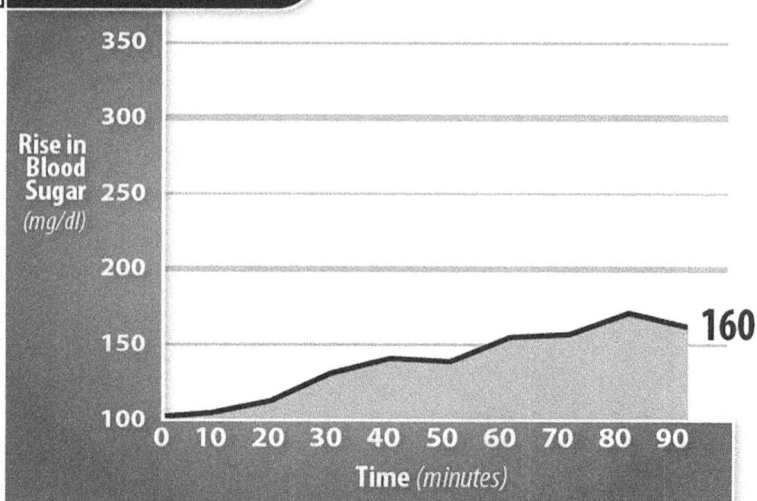

Rise in Blood Sugar (mg/dl)

350
300
250
200
150
100

160

0 10 20 30 40 50 60 70 80 90

Time (minutes)

Total Calories – 87

Oranges

Oranges are in the middle of fruits in terms of blood sugar impact and weight contribution. Not too bad but not as good as the ones to come. I'm a fan of quartering oranges and eating as much of the fiber (what your mom called roughage) as I can.

25 | 20 blackberries

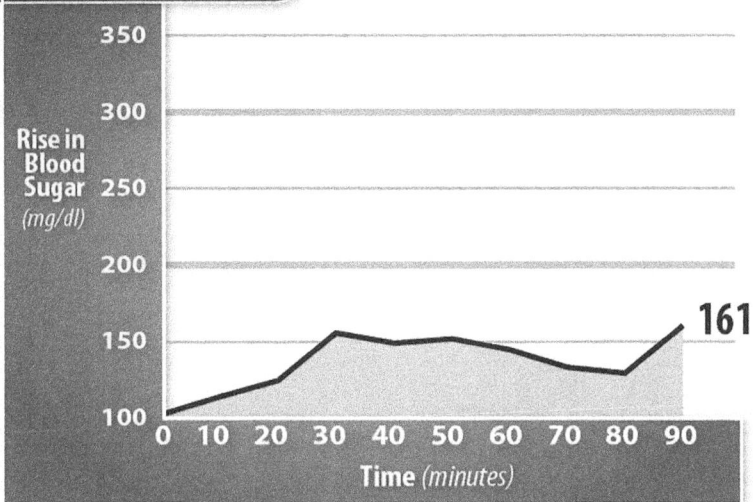

Rise in Blood Sugar (mg/dl)

161

Time (minutes)

Total Calories – 62

Blackberries

Blackberries have about the same impact as oranges. They're not too bad in terms of blood sugar impact but you still won't want to splurge on them.

26 | Medium size apple

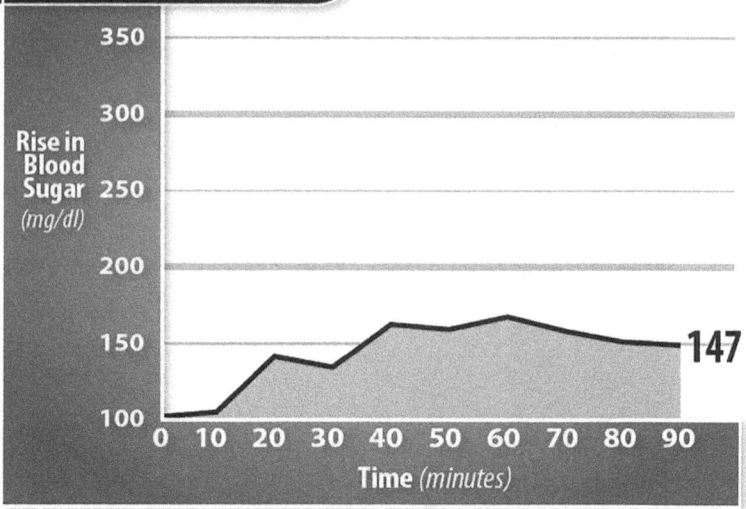

Rise in
Blood
Sugar
(mg/dl)

350
300
250
200
150
100

0 10 20 30 40 50 60 70 80 90

147

Time (minutes)

Total Calories – 95

Apples

Apples are good; not too much impact on blood sugar or weight and not much likelihood of overindulging by eating two or three apples.

27 One cup blueberries

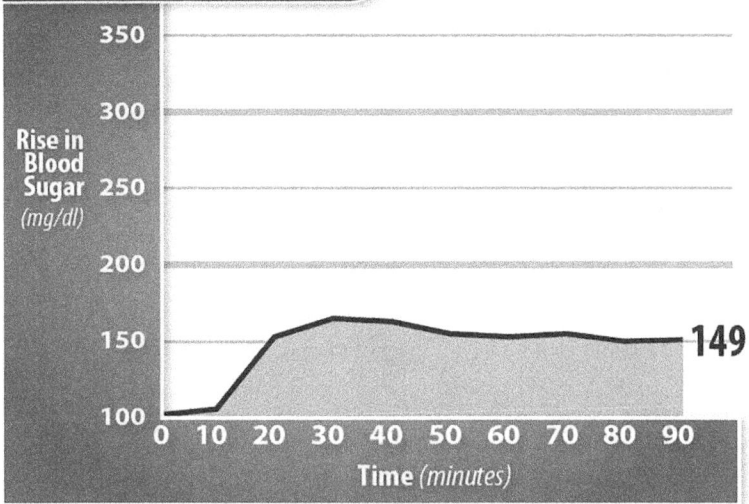

Rise in Blood Sugar 250 *(mg/dl)*

149

Time *(minutes)*

Total Calories – 85

Blueberries

Not only will blueberries have little influence on your blood sugar and weight but everything I've read praises them for all their healthy ingredients.

28 — One large slice cantaloupe

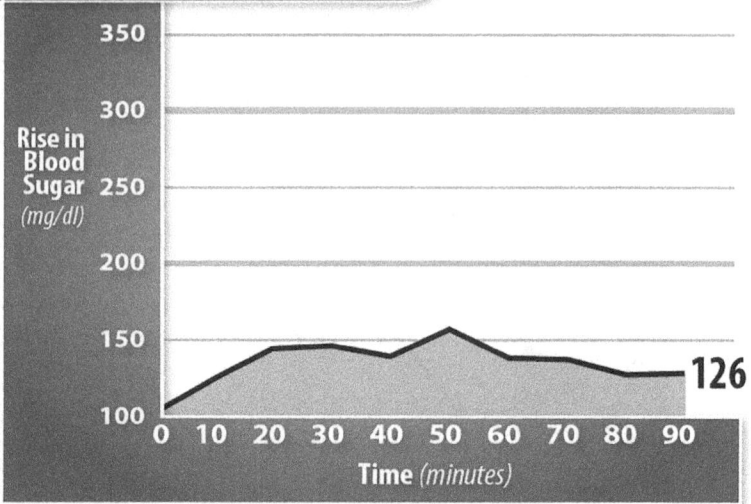

Rise in Blood Sugar (mg/dl)

Time (minutes)

126

Total Calories – 34

Cantaloupe

Cantaloupe in season is one of my favorite breakfast fruits. My helpings are usually moderate and the impact on my blood sugar and weight is very small. This is a fruit that because of its sweet taste, I expected to have a greater impact on my blood sugar than it does.

29 | 1/2 grapefruit *(No sugar added)*

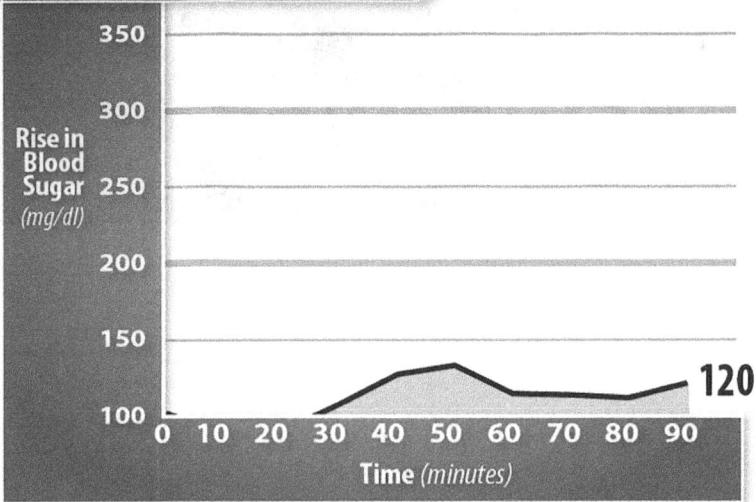

Total Calories – 52

Grapefruit

This graph disagrees with some things I've read about grapefruit causing high rises in blood sugar, but my 30 years of experience with grapefruit is consistent with what this graph shows. By the way, I haven't put sugar on anything since I got diabetes and I don't miss it. I don't use artificial sweeteners on or in anything either because I believe that contributes to maintaining a taste and desire for sweeter things.

Conclusions on the Fruit Carbohydrate Group

Despite the vitamins, minerals, and general health benefits fruits offer, they are not a free ride. In other words, they contribute moderately to increased blood sugar and weight gain. A Type 2 diabetic who is trying to lower blood sugars and anyone trying to lose weight needs to be moderate in the consumption of fruits—especially pineapples, bananas, and cherries.

Fruit Juices

Still within my category of fruit carbohydrates are fruit juices. Following are graphs for three of the most common fruit juices: apple juice, orange juice, and grapefruit juice. I've also tested and graphed my "go-to-juice," V-8, which will give an interesting point of reference.

In the fruit juice graphs, it's important to note how fast the juices increase blood sugar. Because of these fast increases, pay special attention to the volume of the gray area created by the fruit juices as compared to V-8 juice, which has a significantly smaller gray shaded area because of its slower blood sugar increase. It therefore has a much smaller contribution to weight gain. This is a very important concept to grasp. Even if the end point is the same, the slower the rise, the greater the opportunity to burn glucose before it is stored and therefore the less the contribution to weight gain.

30 | 8oz bottle *Minute Maid* apple juice

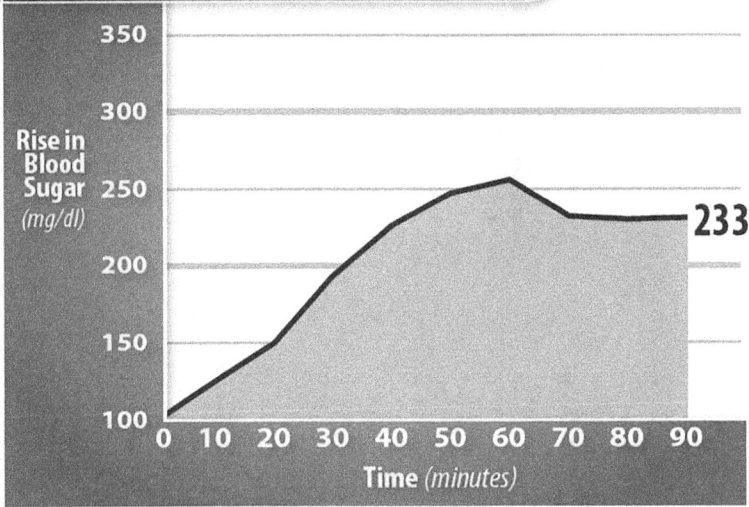

Rise in Blood Sugar *(mg/dl)*

350
300
250
200
150
100

233

0 10 20 30 40 50 60 70 80 90

Time *(minutes)*

Total Calories – 110

Apple Juice

Note that the net blood sugar increase from apple juice is 133 mg/dl. That approaches three times the 47 mg/dl blood sugar increase of a medium-size apple (graph 26). But even more important than that, note the huge difference in the volume of the shaded area of the apple juice compared to an apple. This is a dramatic visualization of the huge contribution to weight increase of the juice compared to the fruit itself.

31 | 8 oz orange juice

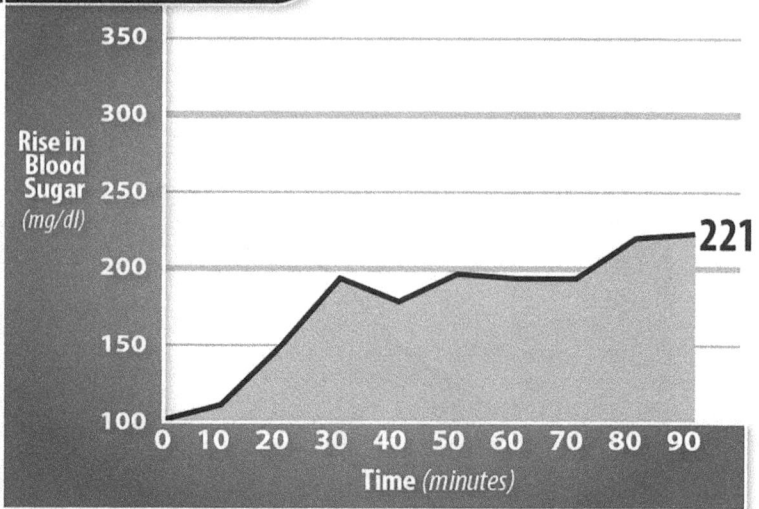

Total Calories – 102

Orange Juice

Orange juice provides a similar comparison though not as dramatic as apple juice. The net rise in blood sugar caused by orange juice is 121 mg/dl compared to 60 for a large orange. Once again though, because the orange juice increases blood sugar so much faster, the shaded area representing the juice's contribution to weight gain is significantly larger than the orange itself.

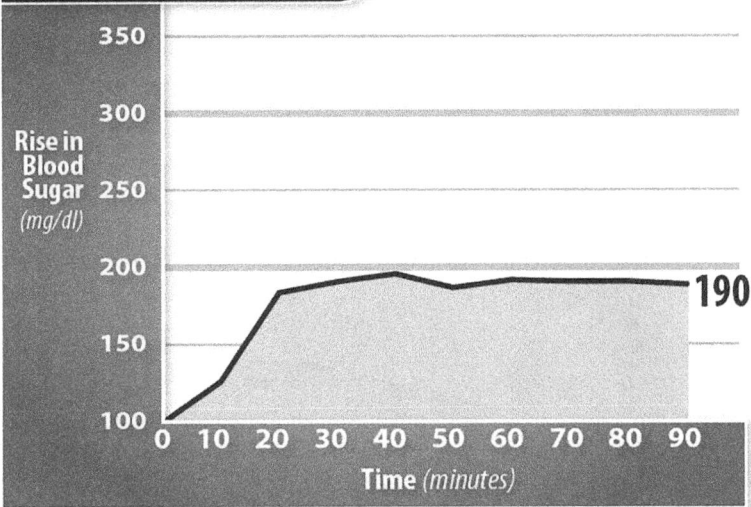

32 | **8 oz Grapefruit juice**

Rise in Blood Sugar (mg/dl)

190

Time (minutes)

Total Calories – 88

Grapefruit Juice

Now compare grapefruit juice to ½ grapefruit (graph 29). Not only does the juice cause a much bigger rise than the grapefruit itself but because it causes such a fast rise, it goes into your bloodstream faster than you can use it and much of the glucose it causes—just like apple juice and orange juice—will end up being stored in the liver or as body fat. This comparison also shows the net blood sugar rise for ½ grapefruit of 20 mg/dl compared to a net rise of the juice of 90. Now some will argue that I should have compared a full grapefruit to 8 ounces of juice. They may be right but my goal here is to compare typical portions. I don't ever recall seeing anyone eating two grapefruit halves in a restaurant but I often see folks drinking 8 ounces or more of whatever juice they ordered. Even if I were to double the grapefruit portion, it would still be less than half the increase in blood sugar of the juice.

33 | 8 oz V8 Juice

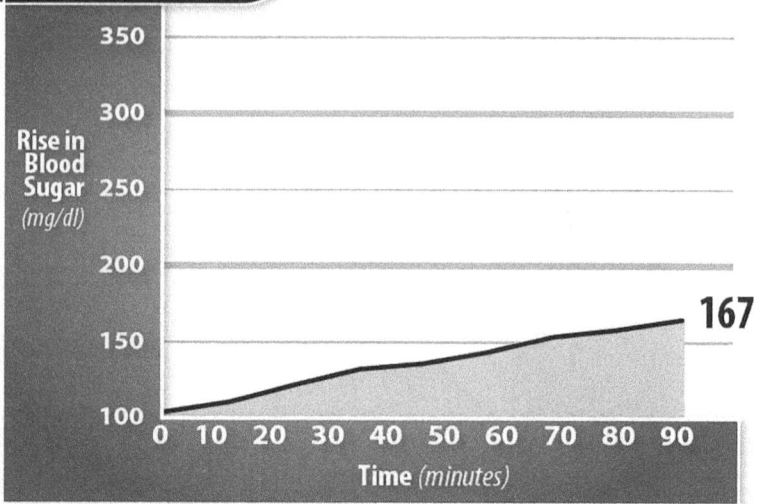

Rise in Blood Sugar (mg/dl)

350
300
250
200
167
150
100

0 10 20 30 40 50 60 70 80 90

Time (minutes)

Total Calories – 50

V-8 Juice

This graph is a good illustration of the value of foods or liquids that cause slower rises in blood sugar. In this case, the V-8 juice reaches the same quite-high level that the other juices do, but it reaches that level much more slowly—over a 90- minute period as shown in these graphs. The very slow rise in glucose means less of the glucose created by V-8 juice will be stored since you'll be burning it as it enters. You won't be able to burn the glucose from the other juices as fast as they go in so the excess glucose will be stored as fat.

I can rarely get V-8 in restaurants but it is the juice of choice for me at home. For the past few years I've been diluting about a third of a large glass of V-8 juice with two thirds of a glass of Pellegrino or Perrier Sparkling Mineral Water. It's now not only my favorite breakfast drink but also a very refreshing midday drink.

Conclusions Regarding Fruit Juices

Diluting your morning fruit juice is one of the easiest actions you can take. The impact on your blood sugar and weight will, of course, depend on how much juice you drink now.

Whether you dilute your juice with mineral water, tap water, or bottled water, you'll soon find the diluted juice becoming an easy and refreshing pattern that will become a habit in no time. It's one of those small actions that will make a big difference over time.

Vegetable Carbohydrates

Now we're getting into the good stuff. Your mother was right—eat your vegetables. She probably told you they would make you healthy but what she didn't know is how little they contribute to blood sugar increases and weight gain. To the extent that you can eat more of the foods that have little impact on your blood sugar and less of the foods that have greater impact on your blood sugar you will lose weight even if you're eating the same volume of food. As you will see, vegetables are the carbohydrate group that has the least impact on your blood sugar.

Take a minute now and go back to the sweet and starchy carbs graphs and compare those to the following veggies carb graphs. Compare how fast sweet and starchy carbs get into your bloodstream, how high they go, and finally, compare the gray area. The faster a food goes in and the higher it goes the greater the gray area and the more weight it's going to add.

34 | 4 Medium Tomato Slices

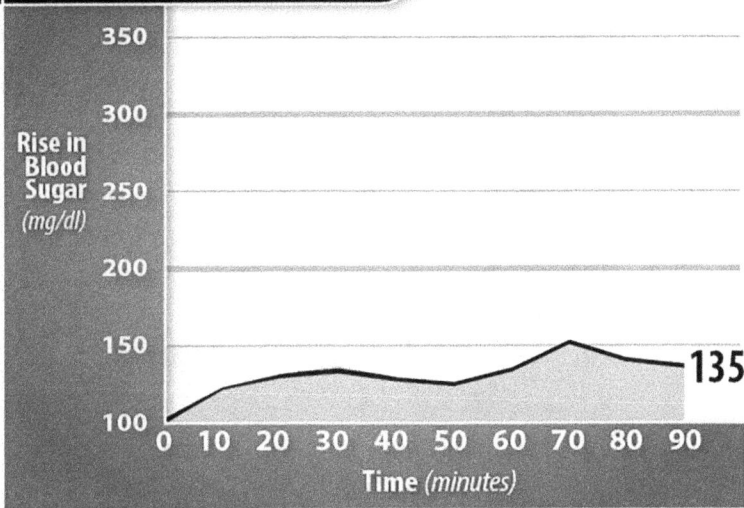

Rise in Blood Sugar (mg/dl)

350
300
250
200
150
135
100

0 10 20 30 40 50 60 70 80 90

Time (minutes)

Total Calories – 20

Tomatoes

Contrary to conventional wisdom, tomatoes are very good for keeping blood sugar and weight down. Be careful of tomato soup, ketchup, and some salsas—all of which often have sugar added.

35 **1 cup cauliflower w/o butter**

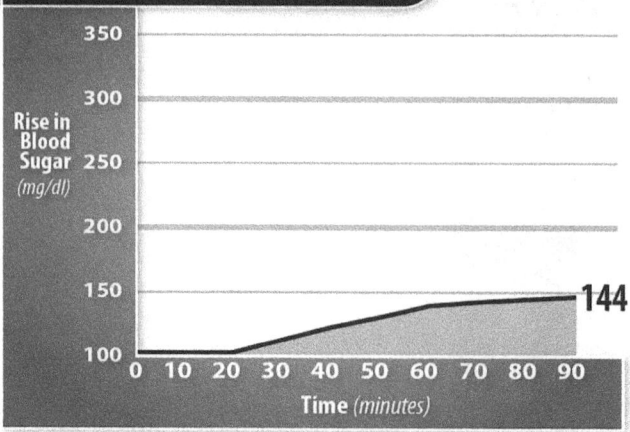

Rise in
Blood
Sugar
(mg/dl)

144

Time (minutes)

Total Calories – 27

36 **One cup cauliflower w/ butter**

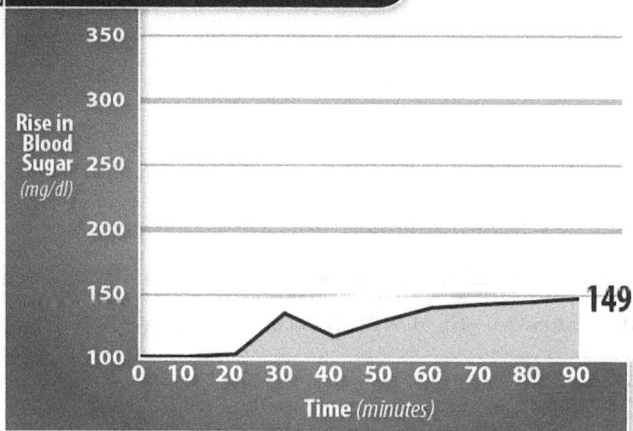

Rise in
Blood
Sugar
(mg/dl)

149

Time (minutes)

Total Calories – 48

Cauliflower

Here's an illustration of a very minor impact of fat (butter) when combined with veggie carbs. You can see by the following two graphs that eating cauliflower with butter creates an almost negligible impact on blood sugar and weight gain.

37 **Asparagus w/ butter**

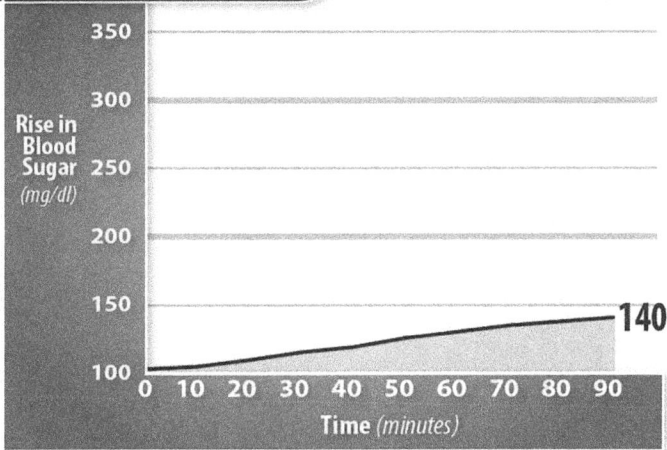

Rise in
Blood
Sugar
(mg/dl)

350
300
250
200
150
140
100

0 10 20 30 40 50 60 70 80 90

Time *(minutes)*

Total Calories – 48

Asparagus

Asparagus with butter has about the same minimal impact on blood sugar and weight as cauliflower with butter.

| 38 | Broccoli w/ butter |

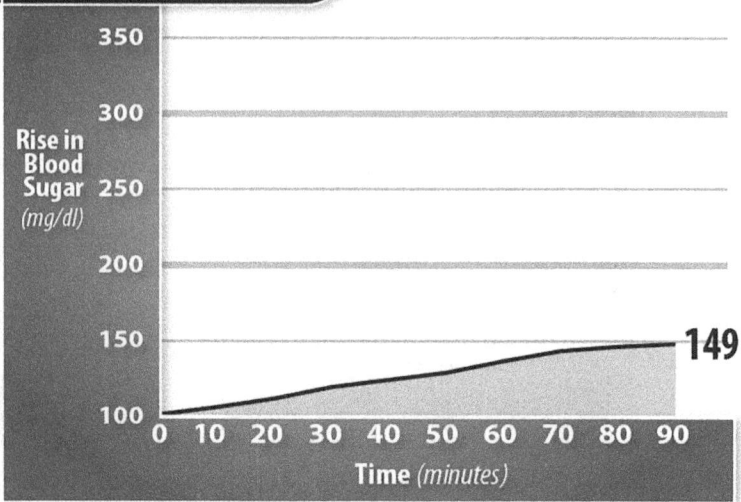

Total Calories – 51

Broccoli

This graph shows broccoli's insignificant impact on blood sugar and weight gain. When I discovered the small impact of putting butter on vegetables, I began eating more vegetables. You will probably eat more vegetables too. It's a good example of eating more of the good foods and less of the bad foods.

A logical question at this point is, "What about the impact this extra butter has on cholesterol levels. I'll respond to that question in the next chapter.

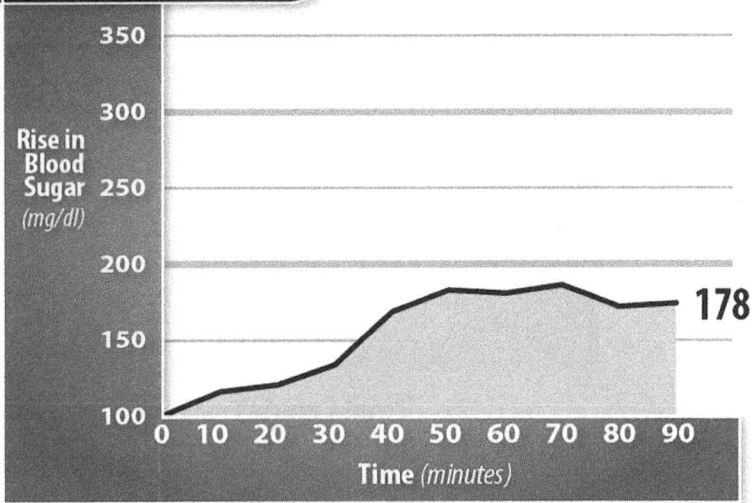

39 **Carrots w/ butter**

Rise in Blood Sugar (mg/dl)

178

Time (minutes)

Total Calories – 71

Carrots

You can see by the graph that the impact of carrots on blood sugar and weight is slightly higher than that of the previous vegetables, but not as high as that of corn and potatoes.

40 | **Corn on the cob (1.5 ears)**

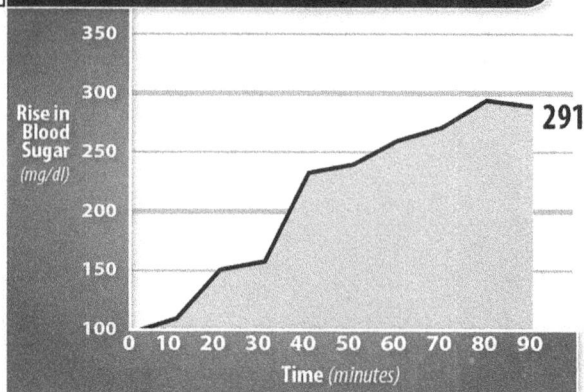

Rise in Blood Sugar (mg/dl)

350
300
250
200
150
100

291

0 10 20 30 40 50 60 70 80 90

Time (minutes)

Total Calories – 232.5

Corn

When I said, "With just a few exceptions, eat more vegetables and you'll lose weight," corn is one of those exceptions. Although corn is considered a vegetable carbohydrate, it acts more like a starchy carbohydrate. Take a look at this graph and compare it to the other veggie carbs. Like starchy carbs, corn creates a lot of blood glucose and therefore insulin demand, which means more weight gain.

Minimize corn in your eating lifestyle.

Like corn, potatoes also act more like a starchy carb than a veggie carb. They are a good source of vitamin C and potassium but are also big contributors to increased blood sugar and therefore weight.

41 **Vegetable Medley w/ Butter**

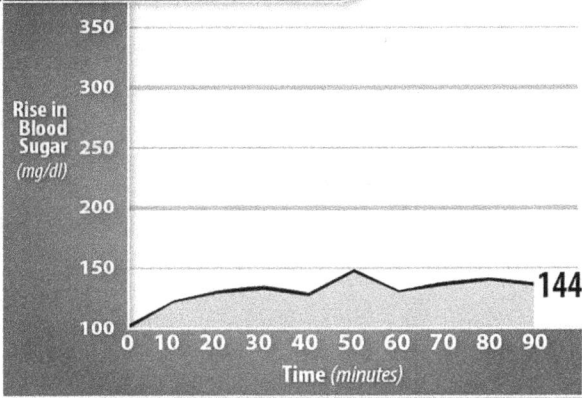

Rise in
Blood
Sugar
(mg/dl)

350
300
250
200
150
100

144

0 10 20 30 40 50 60 70 80 90

Time (minutes)

Total Calories – 125

This vegetable medley consists of broccoli, cauliflower, and carrots

Conclusions on Vegetable Carbohydrate Group

A very important message from these graphs is that vegetables in general have very little impact on blood sugar and weight gain and put very little pressure on the pancreas to produce more insulin.

Adding butter to vegetables has only a tiny impact on blood sugar.

Because neither vegetables nor fat trigger much insulin demand, the mixture of vegetables and butter in the stomach allows only a very limited amount of those combined calories to get into the cells for storage as fat.

This is different from adding butter to starchy carbs, which—as you've now seen—triggers a lot of insulin demand. All the insulin created by the starchy carbs allows the butter calories to flow into storage cells since the two items are mixed together in the stomach.

I've had so many people tell me that reducing the quantity of food they eat is very difficult and they always feel hungry. One way to solve that problem and lose weight is to eat more of the foods that don't raise your blood sugar much and less of the foods that do. That means eat more vegetables and be free with the butter.

Protein and Fat

I've combined protein and fat because very few common foods are exclusively fat. The two most common foods that derive all their calories from fat are butter (100 calories per serving—all from fat) and olive oil (125 calories per serving—all from fat). Wow, with those calories from fat, they must be bad for you. Right? ... I think you'll be surprised!

Once again compare the upcoming graphs to the big increases in blood sugar caused by sweet carbs, starchy carbs, and fruit juices.

First some breakfast foods containing both protein and fat.

42 **Three large fried eggs**

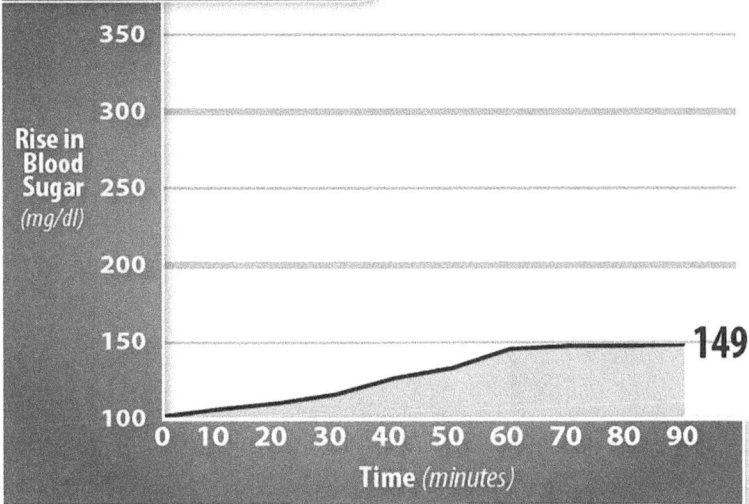

Rise in Blood Sugar (mg/dl)

149

Time (minutes)

Total Calories – 276

43 **Three large poached eggs**

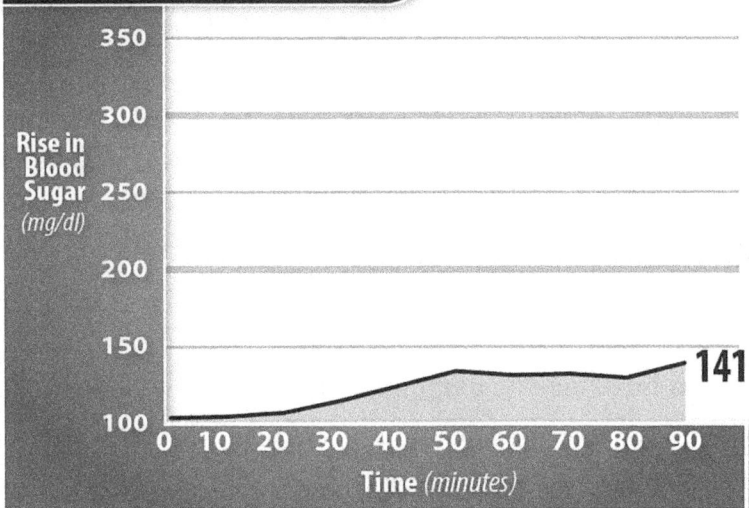

Rise in Blood Sugar (mg/dl)

141

Time (minutes)

Total Calories – 213

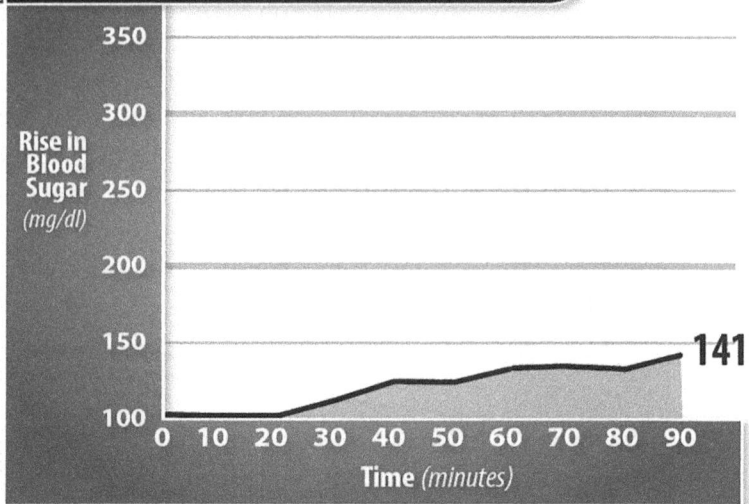

44 | **3 Soft Boiled Eggs w/ Butter**

Rise in Blood Sugar (mg/dl) — 141

Time (minutes)

Total Calories – 234

Three Large Eggs

Large eggs have 70 calories each so three eggs have 210 calories, exactly the same number of calories as a Hershey bar (also 210 calories). Now compare the graphs—a Hershey bar (graph 4) to the next two graphs, three large eggs (graphs 42, 43, and 44). It very strongly illustrates the point that calories are not always a good indicator of the impact on blood sugar or weight creation. Take special note of the area of gray under the graphs, which you know by now is a general representation of weight gain.

It's a good illustration of the value of foods that enter your bloodstream more slowly. Remember, the slower the food enters your bloodstream, the more likely you'll burn it before you store it. You'll also note very little difference between poached eggs and boiled or fried eggs. The boiled and fried eggs include butter and the poached eggs don't—thus the difference in calories but the gain in blood sugar and weight gain despite the increase in calories is insignificant.

Bacon

I'm very sure this is going to be one of your biggest surprises. It took me decades to figure out why sometimes bacon seemed to have negligible impact on my blood sugar and sometimes it seemed to have a lot of impact. I finally figured out what created the discrepancy.

After thousands of blood sugar tests, I stumbled upon the answer to the discrepancy. About 10 years ago I started periodically eating breakfasts with just bacon and eggs or sausage and eggs—no potatoes or toast. I was stunned at how little impact that combination, without toast, pancakes, or potatoes had on my blood sugar. I gave myself less insulin for those breakfasts and started losing weight without even trying to.

Since then I have learned that I can add almost any vegetable—with butter—to that combination of bacon and eggs or just eggs and similar blood-sugar-lowering, and weight loss will result.

Compare the bacon graph to the single piece of wheat toast with and without butter (graphs 19 and 20). That comparison provides a good example of the relative contribution to your weight of toast vs. bacon.

Now few people eat bacon alone; I sure don't. So following this section on protein and fat, you'll find a section titled, "Good Meals, Bad meals" which will show you which combinations of foods will trigger high blood sugar and weight gain and which will trigger lower blood sugars and weight loss.

So if fat's not the problem, and starchy carbs are, how about heart health and cholesterol? I cover this in more detail in the next chapter.

45 | Two large bacon slices

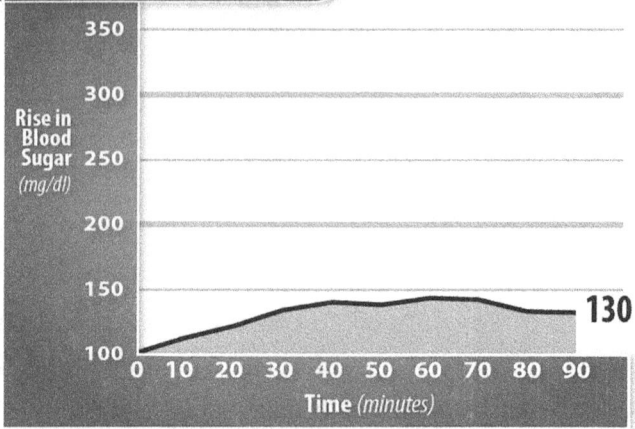

Rise in Blood Sugar (mg/dl)

350
300
250
200
150
130
100

0 10 20 30 40 50 60 70 80 90
Time (minutes)

Total Calories – 86

46 | Two Pork Sausage Patties

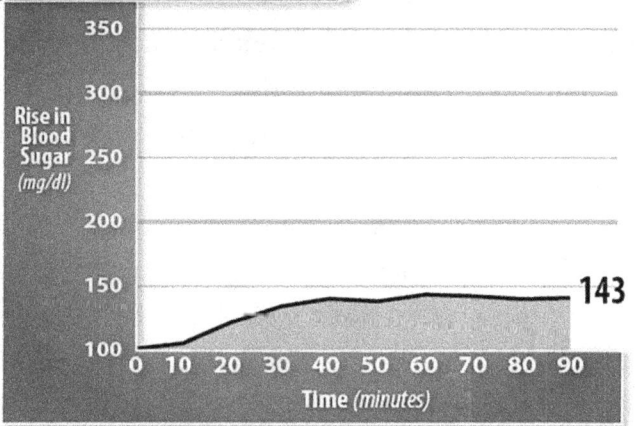

Rise in Blood Sugar (mg/dl)

350
300
250
200
150
143
100

0 10 20 30 40 50 60 70 80 90
Time (minutes)

Total Calories – 290

47 | **8 oz Ribeye steak**

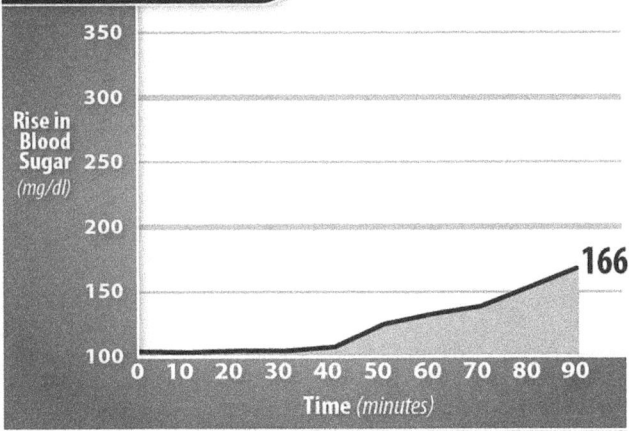

Rise in
Blood
Sugar
(mg/dl)

350
300
250
200
150 — **166**
100

0 10 20 30 40 50 60 70 80 90
Time *(minutes)*

Total Calories – 480

48 | **Rotisserie chicken with skin (three pieces)**

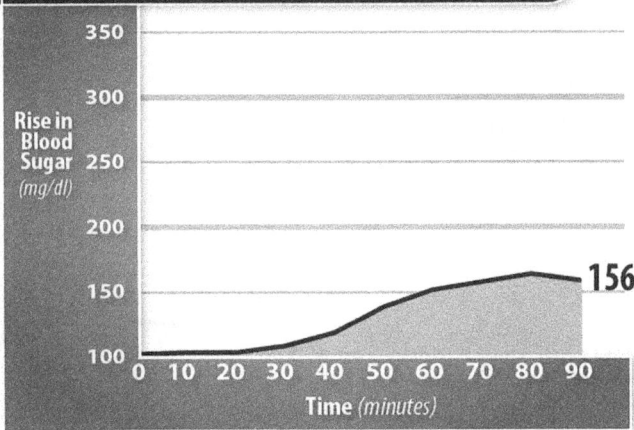

Rise in
Blood
Sugar
(mg/dl)

350
300
250
200
150 — **156**
100

0 10 20 30 40 50 60 70 80 90
Time *(minutes)*

Total Calories – 330

Rib-Eye Steak and Rotisserie Chicken

Rib-eye steak and rotisserie chicken are two more examples of the low blood sugar impact of protein and fat if not combined with starchy carbs. The skin is not a problem but later you'll see that breading is.

49 **8 oz grilled halibut**

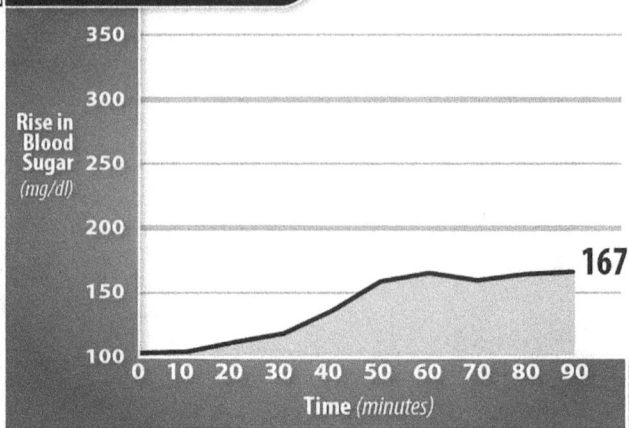

Rise in
Blood
Sugar
(mg/dl)

350
300
250
200
167
150
100

0 10 20 30 40 50 60 70 80 90

Time (minutes)

Total Calories – 249

50 **10 oz grilled salmon**

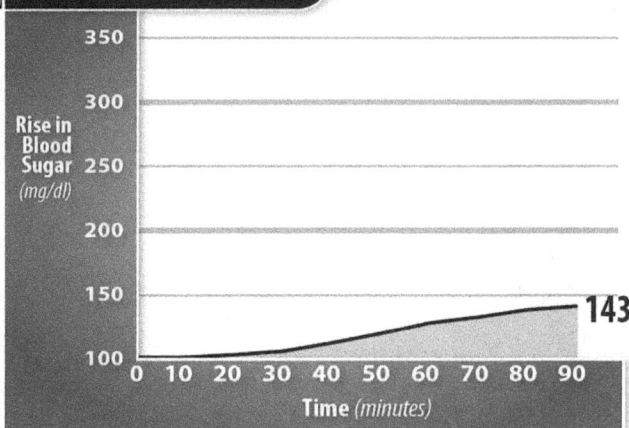

Rise in
Blood
Sugar
(mg/dl)

350
300
250
200
150
143
100

0 10 20 30 40 50 60 70 80 90

Time (minutes)

Total Calories – 402

Halibut and Salmon

Both of these cold-water fish are excellent choices to keep blood sugar and weight down. In the next group of graphs for "Good Meals, Bad Meals" you'll see how meals with these two fish choices plus Pacific cod can contribute to lowering blood sugar and losing weight.

51 | 1 Slice Provolone Cheese

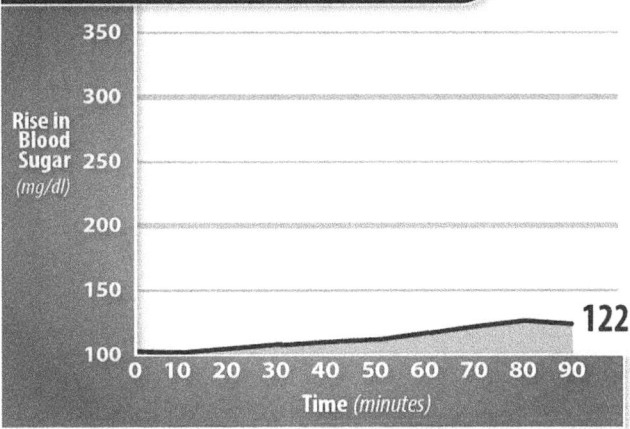

Rise in Blood Sugar *(mg/dl)*

350
300
250
200
150
100

122

0 10 20 30 40 50 60 70 80 90

Time *(minutes)*

Total Calories – 100

52 | 1 Serving Reg. Cottage Cheese

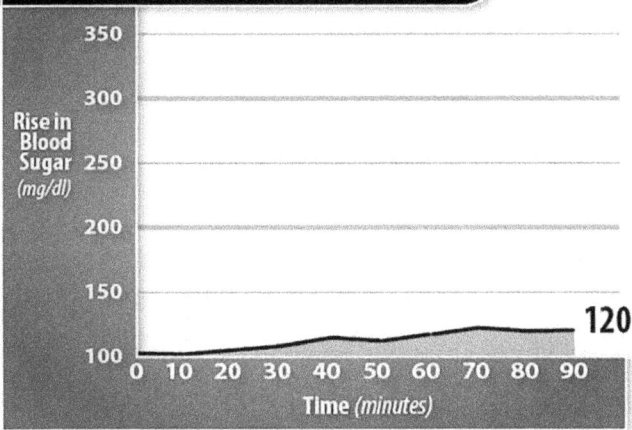

Rise in Blood Sugar *(mg/dl)*

350
300
250
200
150
100

120

0 10 20 30 40 50 60 70 80 90

Time *(minutes)*

Total Calories – 222

53 | 2 Slices Med. Cheddar Cheese

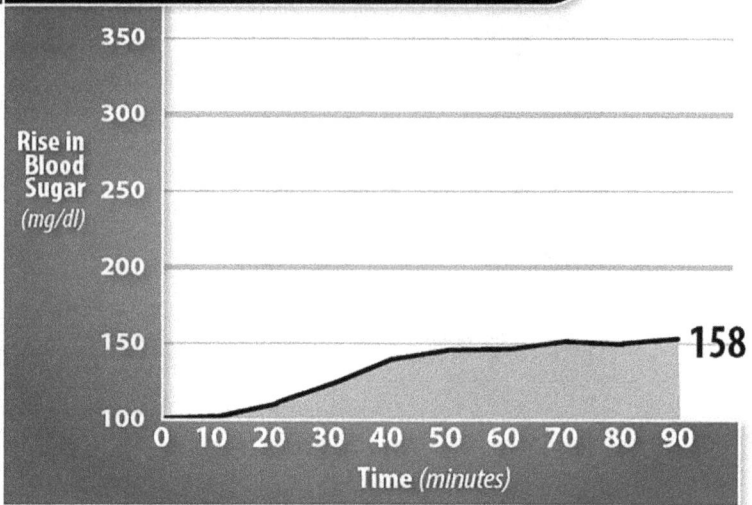

Rise in Blood Sugar (mg/dl)

350
300
250
200
150 ——— **158**
100

0 10 20 30 40 50 60 70 80 90

Time *(minutes)*

Total Calories – 200

Cheeses

Most cheese has little impact on blood sugar and weight. They provide a good snack or addition to a meal. I often put a small amount of cheese in a microwave for 30 seconds and melt it and eat it alone—without crackers or chips—for an evening snack. Notice the small impact of cottage cheese despite the relatively big number of calories.

54 | 1 Serving Cashews (40 pieces)

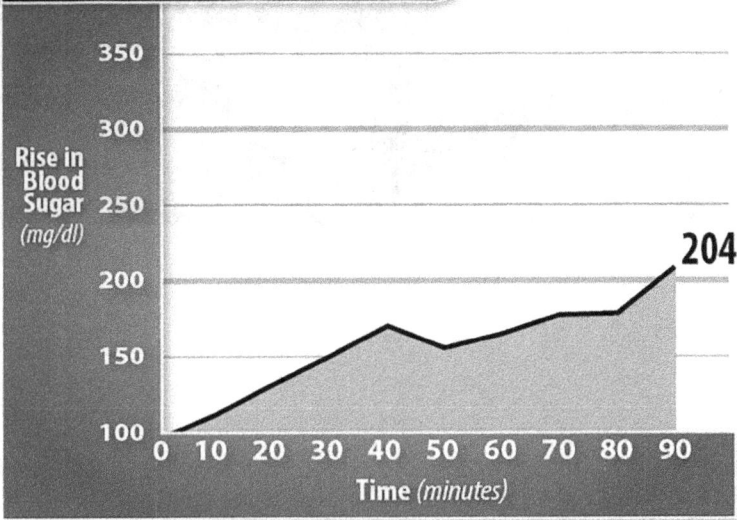

204

Rise in Blood Sugar (mg/dl)

Time (minutes)

Total Calories – 157

Cashews and Almonds

As you can see by this graph of cashews, they don't raise blood sugar by a lot but they are not a free ride. This reflects the impact of 40 cashews which the label says is a "serving." I recommend half that many as a better snack size. Shaved almonds baked on a flat pan and salted make a good-tasting and healthy snack.

Good Meals, Bad Meals

We don't just eat individual foods; we combine them and create meals. You now know that sweet carbs and starchy carbs cause big rises in blood sugar and are big contributors to weight gain. In the following groups of meals, pay close attention to which of the meals have starchy carbs in them and which don't, then note their comparative impacts on blood sugar and therefore on weight gain.I realize that having vegetables with eggs for breakfast is a huge shift in eating lifestyles for most Americans. But if you really care about lowering blood sugar, losing weight, and living a longer, healthier life; breakfast is a good place to start and adding vegetables is a good way to start. Compare these breakfast graphs (55–60) to the next four breakfast graphs (61–64), which all have some starchy carbs in them. That should provide some motivation to eliminate starchy carbs and include vegetable carbs in your breakfasts, plus, you really do have a wide variety of vegetables from which to choose.

Once again these graphs show that the type of food you eat is much more important than the calories in determining blood sugar increases and weight gain.

55 Five egg white vegetable omelette

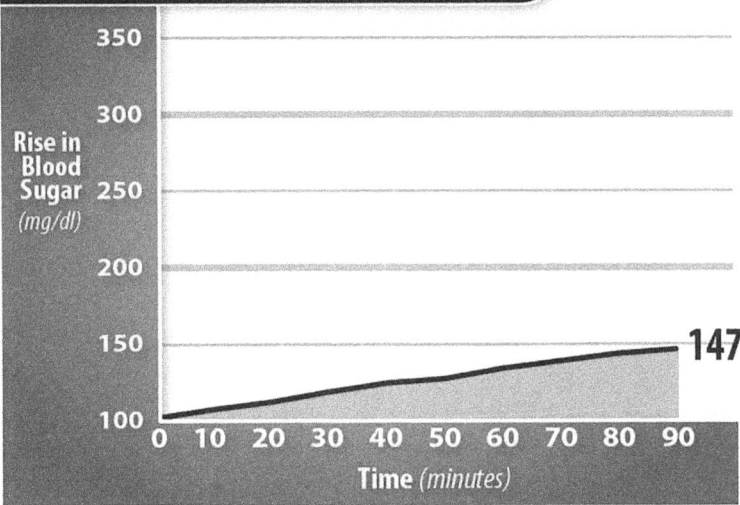

Rise in Blood Sugar *(mg/dl)*

350
300
250
200
150 **147**
100

0 10 20 30 40 50 60 70 80 90
Time *(minutes)*

Total Calories – 110

56 Two eggs, cauliflower w/ butter

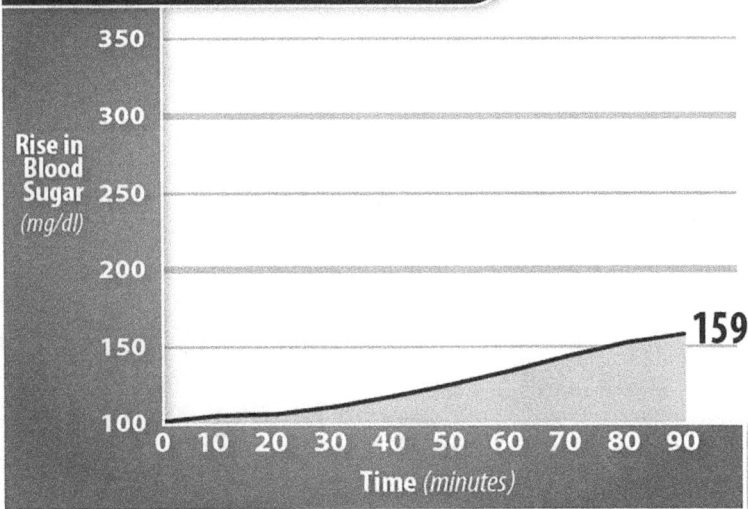

Rise in Blood Sugar *(mg/dl)*

350
300
250
200
150 **159**
100

0 10 20 30 40 50 60 70 80 90
Time *(minutes)*

Total Calories – 230

57 | Two eggs, broccoli w/ butter

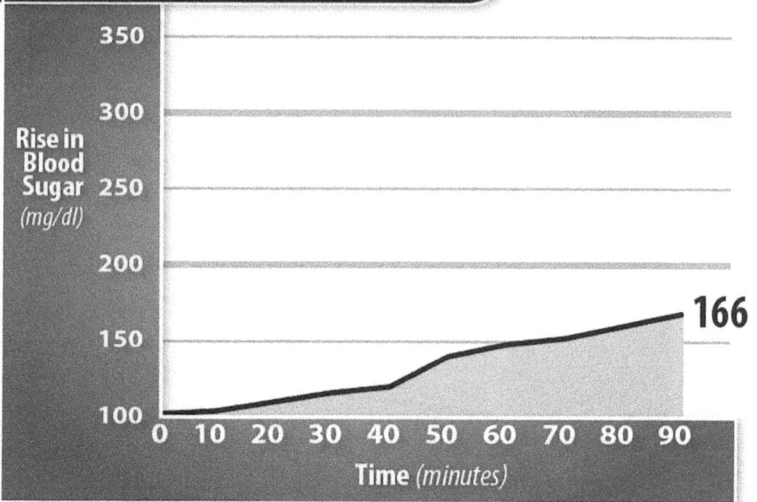

Rise in Blood Sugar (mg/dl)

350
300
250
200
150
100

166

Time (minutes)
0 10 20 30 40 50 60 70 80 90

Total Calories – 233

58 | 2 Fried Eggs & 2 Slices Bacon

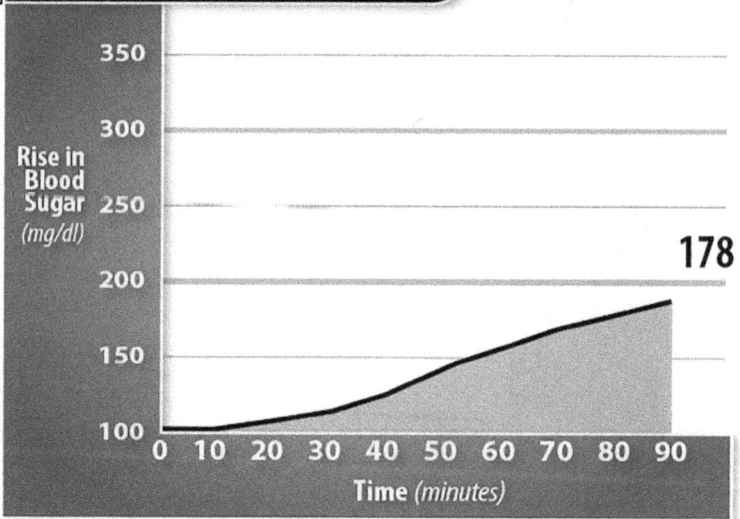

Rise in Blood Sugar (mg/dl)

350
300
250
200
150
100

178

Time (minutes)
0 10 20 30 40 50 60 70 80 90

Total Calories – 266

59 | 3 Fried Eggs, Ground Sirloin, Tomato Slices

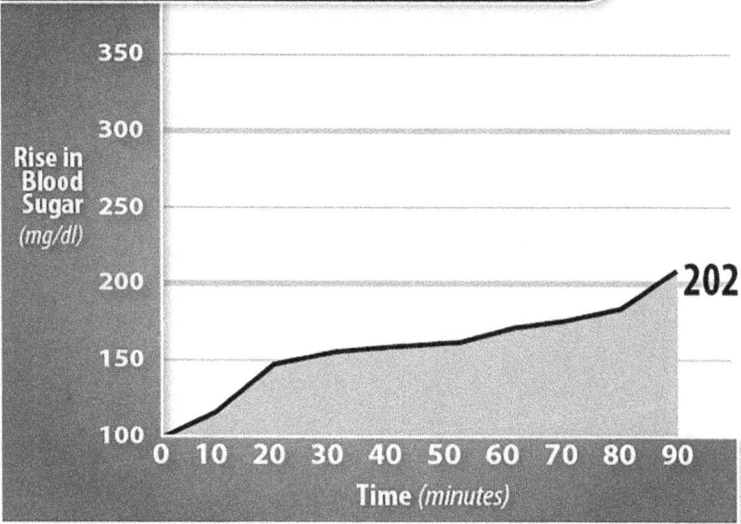

Rise in Blood Sugar (mg/dl)

350
300
250
200 — **202**
150
100

0 10 20 30 40 50 60 70 80 90
Time (minutes)

Total Calories – 502

60 | 2 Fried Eggs & 10 oz Ground Beef

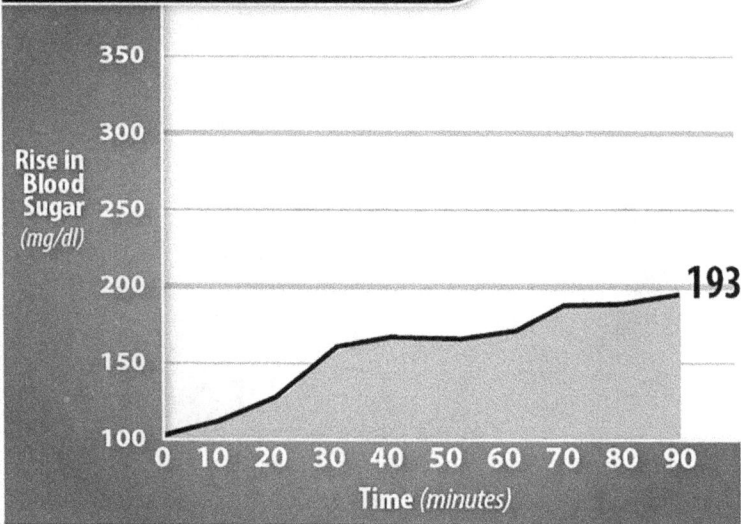

Rise in Blood Sugar (mg/dl)

350
300
250
200
150 — **193**
100

0 10 20 30 40 50 60 70 80 90
Time (minutes)

Total Calories – 1,121

61 Two eggs, hash browns, wheat toast w/ butter

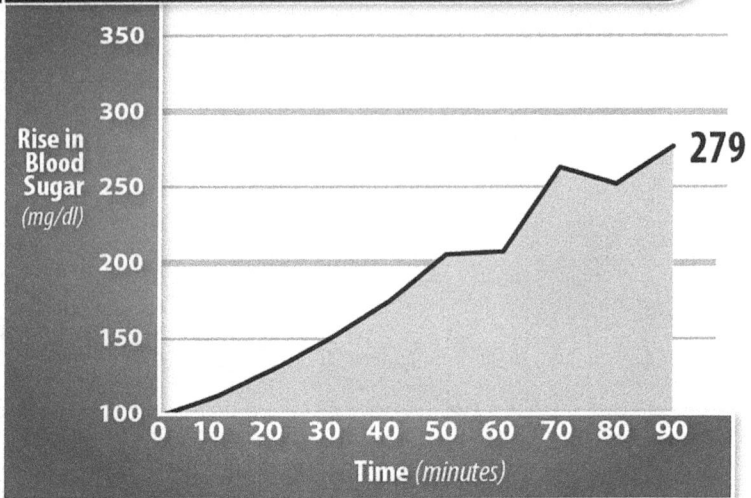

Rise in Blood Sugar *(mg/dl)*

279

Time *(minutes)*

Total Calories – 742

62 One cup *Total* with blueberries and skim milk
(No sugar added)

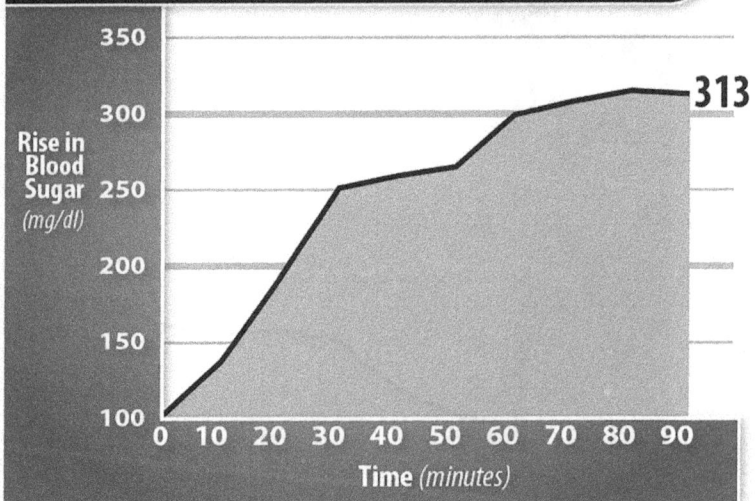

Rise in Blood Sugar *(mg/dl)*

313

Time *(minutes)*

Total Calories – 232

63 Three eggs, sausage, potatoes, wheat toast

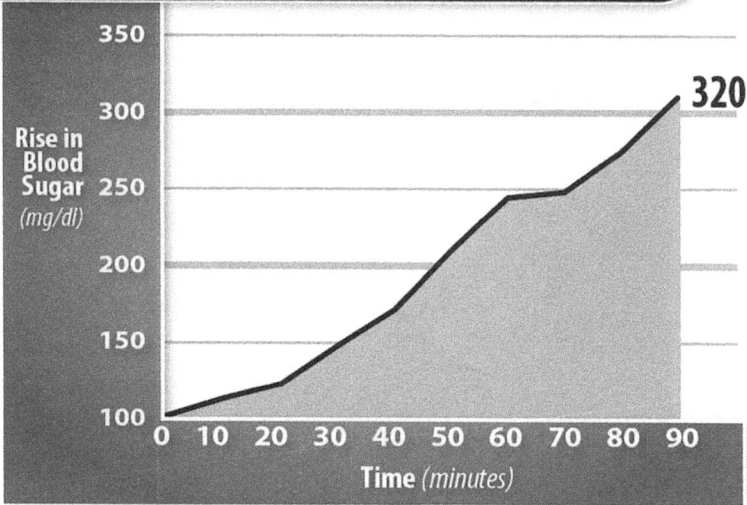

Rise in Blood Sugar *(mg/dl)*

320

Time *(minutes)*

Total Calories – 687

64 Sausage links, two eggs, two pancakes

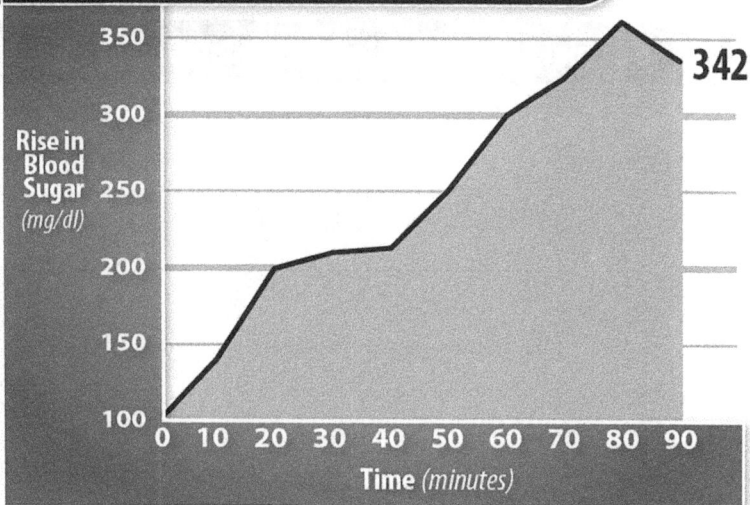

Rise in Blood Sugar *(mg/dl)*

342

Time *(minutes)*

Total Calories – 761

65 | *Egg McMuffin & Hashbrowns*

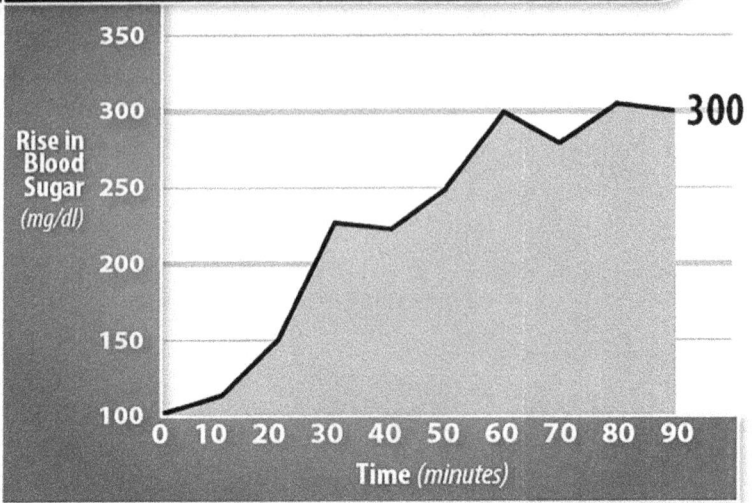

Rise in Blood Sugar *(mg/dl)*

Time *(minutes)*

300

Total Calories – 460

66 | 6 oz filet, vegetables, lettuce wedge w/ blue cheese

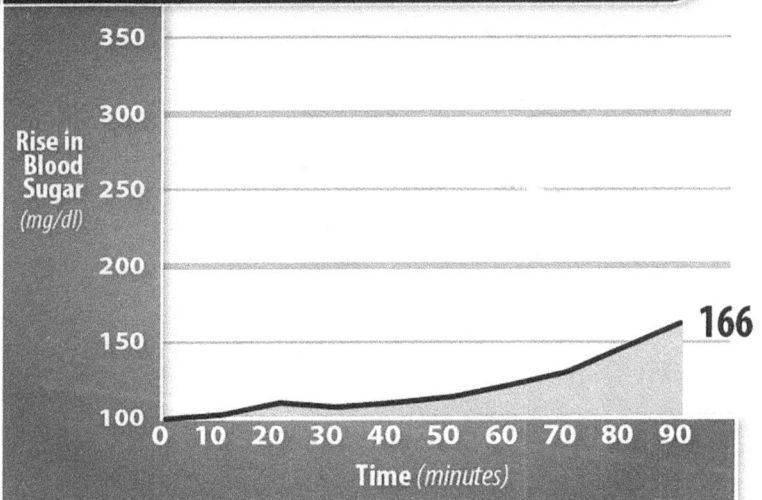

Rise in Blood Sugar *(mg/dl)*

Time *(minutes)*

166

Total Calories – 692

67 Roasted chicken, tomatoes, avacados, salad

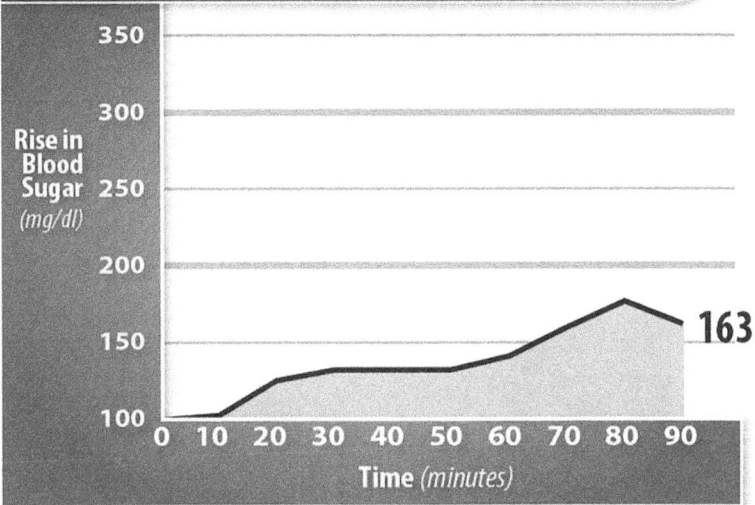

Rise in Blood Sugar *(mg/dl)*

350
300
250
200
150
100

163

0 10 20 30 40 50 60 70 80 90
Time *(minutes)*

Total Calories – 413

68 8 oz Ribeye steak, broccoli, butter, cottage cheese

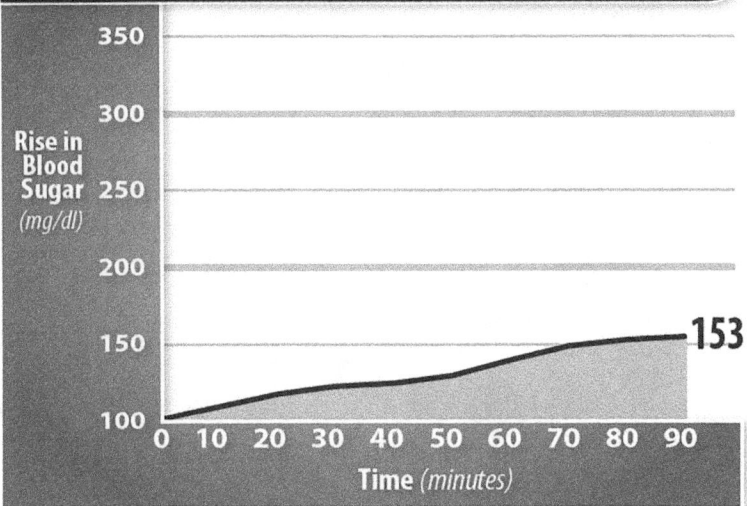

Rise in Blood Sugar *(mg/dl)*

350
300
250
200
150
100

153

0 10 20 30 40 50 60 70 80 90
Time *(minutes)*

Total Calories – 1,120

69 | Grilled Halibut & Broccoli w/Butter

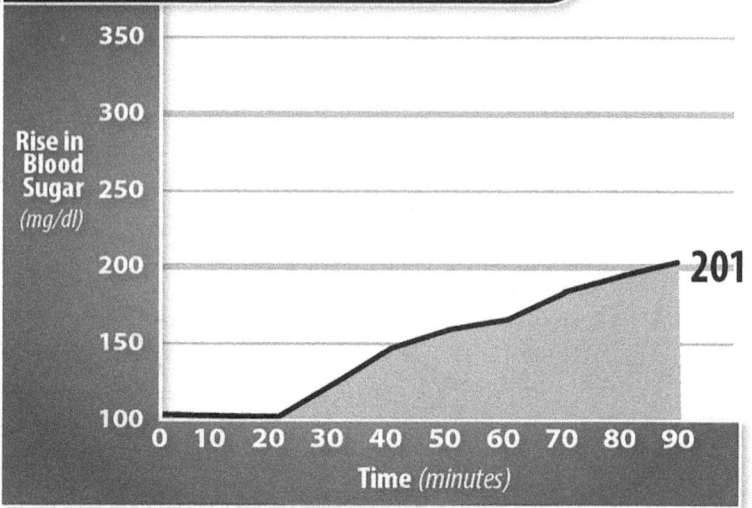

Rise in Blood Sugar *(mg/dl)*

Time *(minutes)*

201

Total Calories – 453

70 | Crab, broccoli, butter

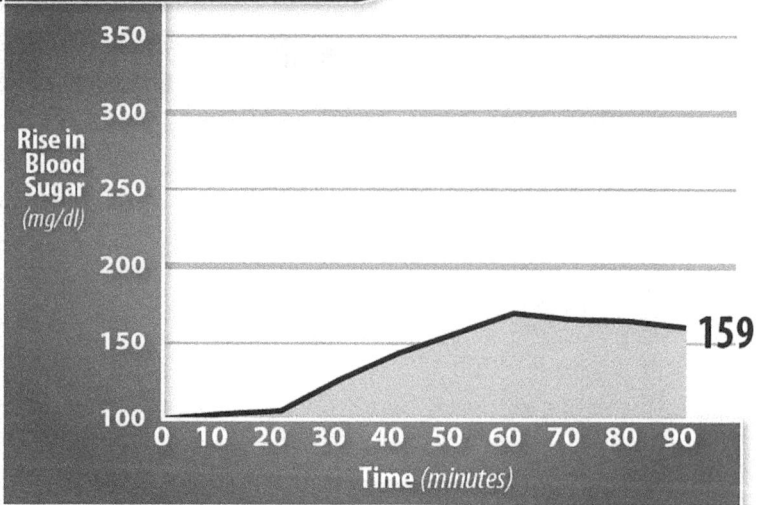

Rise in Blood Sugar *(mg/dl)*

Time *(minutes)*

159

Total Calories – 396

71 — Blackened salmon, brocolli, salad

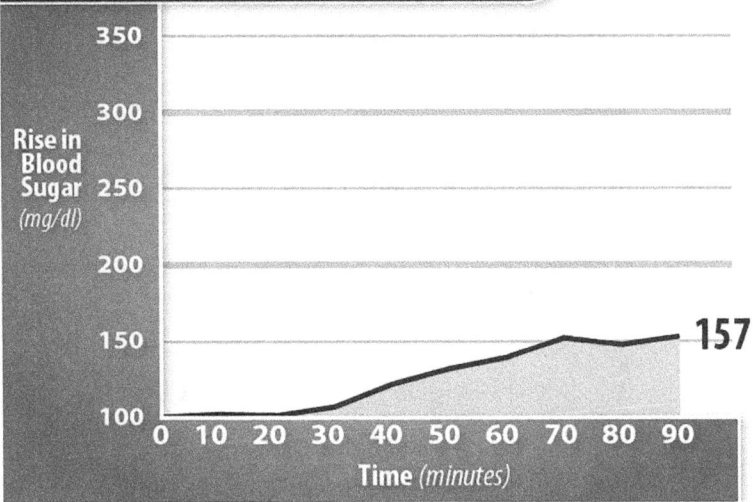

Rise in
Blood
Sugar
(mg/dl)

350
300
250
200
150
100

157

Time *(minutes)*
0 10 20 30 40 50 60 70 80 90

Total Calories – 336

72 — 10 oz. cod w/ butter, cauliflower, green salad

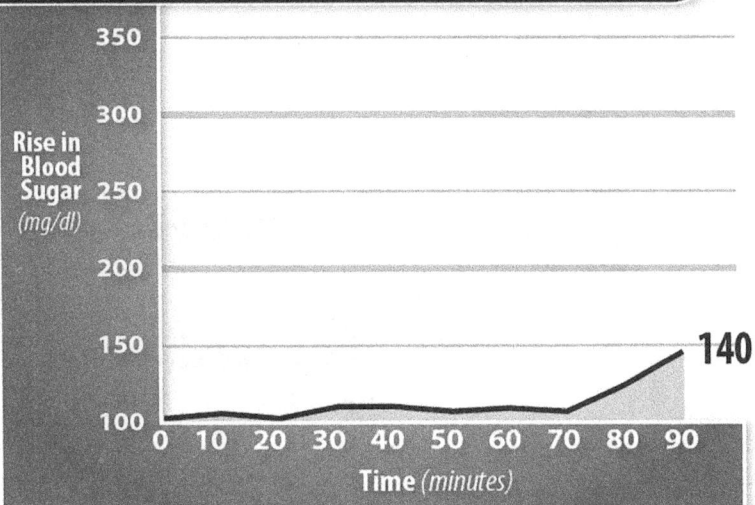

Rise in
Blood
Sugar
(mg/dl)

350
300
250
200
150
100

140

Time *(minutes)*
0 10 20 30 40 50 60 70 80 90

Total Calories – 291

73 Shrimp, asparagus, salad (oil & vinegar dressing)

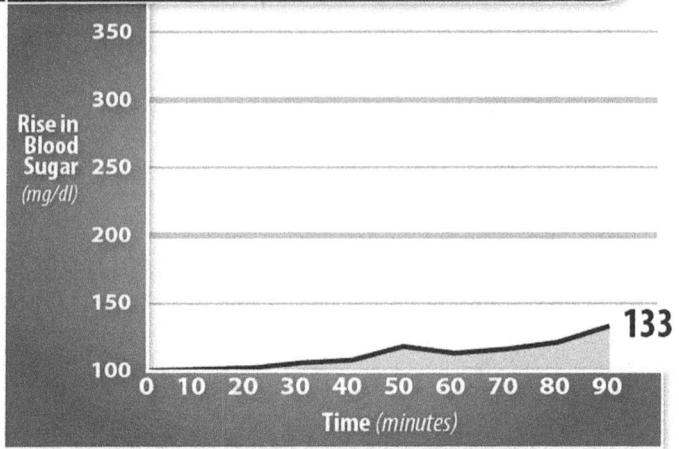

Rise in Blood Sugar (mg/dl)

350
300
250
200
150
100

0 10 20 30 40 50 60 70 80 90

Time (minutes)

133

Total Calories – 140

74 *Carl's Jr.* 1/3lb Low Carb Burger

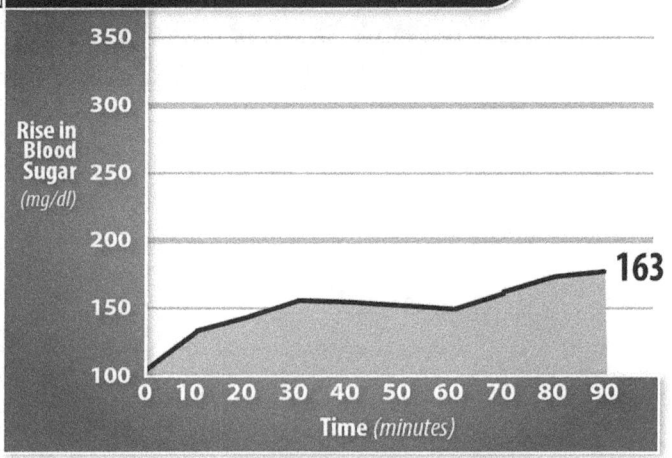

Rise in Blood Sugar (mg/dl)

350
300
250
200
150
100

0 10 20 30 40 50 60 70 80 90

Time (minutes)

163

Total Calories – 450

75 | 8oz Ribeye, Baked Potato, Bread

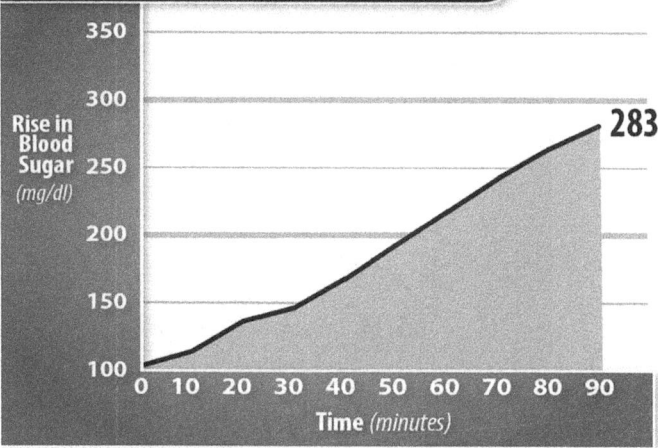

Rise in Blood Sugar *(mg/dl)*

283

Time *(minutes)*

Total Calories – 618

76 | Pasta, marinara sauce, garlic toast, olive oil

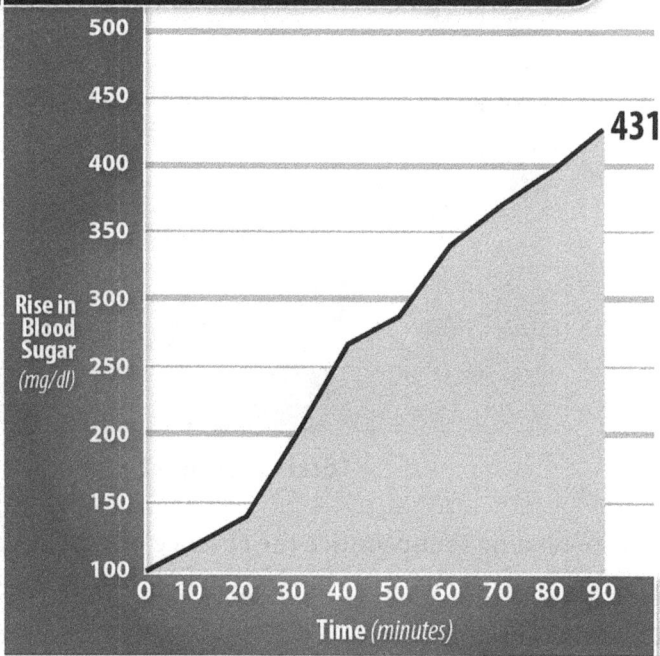

Rise in Blood Sugar *(mg/dl)*

431

Time *(minutes)*

Total Calories – 780

77 Cheeseburger and fries

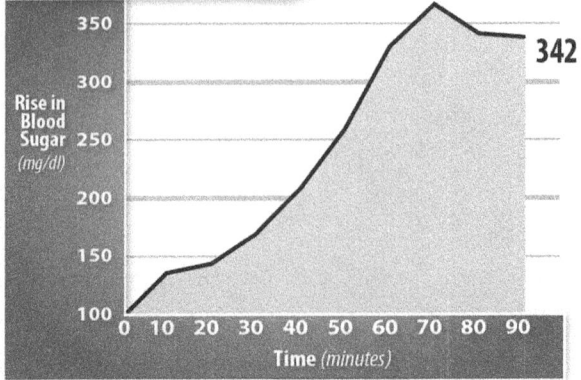

Rise in Blood Sugar (mg/dl)

342

Time (minutes)

Total Calories – 668

78 Three pieces extra crunchy chicken, mashed potatoes, corn, biscuit

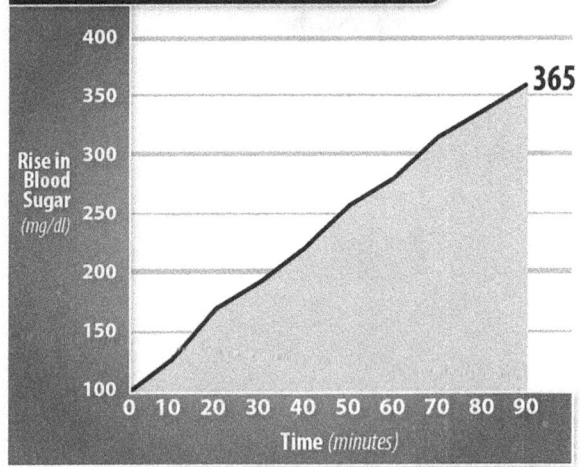

Rise in Blood Sugar (mg/dl)

365

Time (minutes)

Total Calories – 1,600

With the preceding group, notice the absence of starchy carbs. Now compare these graphs with the following High-Blood-Sugar, Weight-Gain Dinners Graphs.

In graph 78, note that it's not just skin on the chicken but it is breading. Skin is not a problem but breading is.

Yogurt

I don't eat much yogurt but my testing of original vs. nonfat yogurt further illustrates my conclusions that "it's not fat that makes people fat. It's starchy and sweet carbohydrates." Low-fat or no-fat yogurts always list fewer calories and less fat than original or traditional yogurts. So it must mean that low-fat or no-fat yogurts will create less blood sugar increase and less weight gain. Right? No. Wrong! Take a look.

So why do these graphs show that you'll gain more weight with no-fat yogurt than with original yogurt even though the no-fat and low-fat varieties have fewer calories?

It's because the no-fat and low-fat varieties have more sweet or starchy carbs to compensate for the taste given up by taking out the fat. If they take out the 9-calorie-per-gram fat and replace it with 5-calorie-per-gram carbs, the calories will go down. But the issue is not the number of calories, it's the type of food. These graphs illustrate beautifully that more sweet and starchy carbs and less fat is the problem. Fewer carbs and more fat is the solution. Give up that chalky, bad-tasting, no-fat yogurt and enjoy the better-tasting original or traditional yogurt.

79 Oikos traditional Greek yogurt

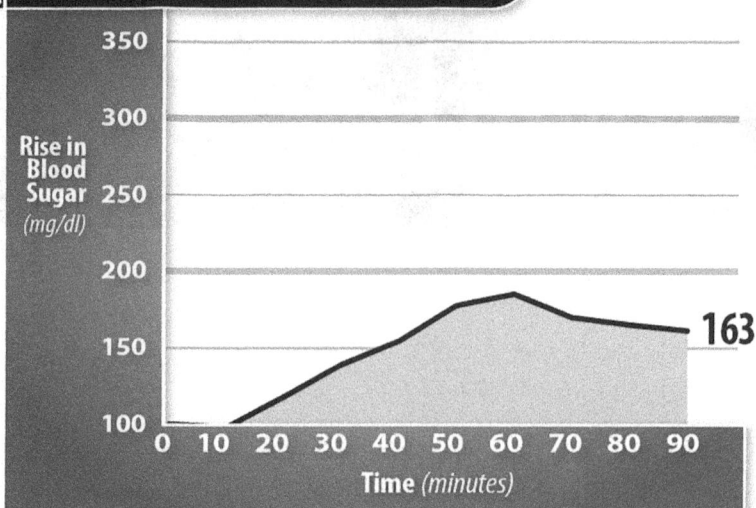

Rise in Blood Sugar (mg/dl)

350
300
250
200
150
100

0 10 20 30 40 50 60 70 80 90

163

Time (minutes)

Total Calories – 63

80 Oikos Greek non-fat yogurt

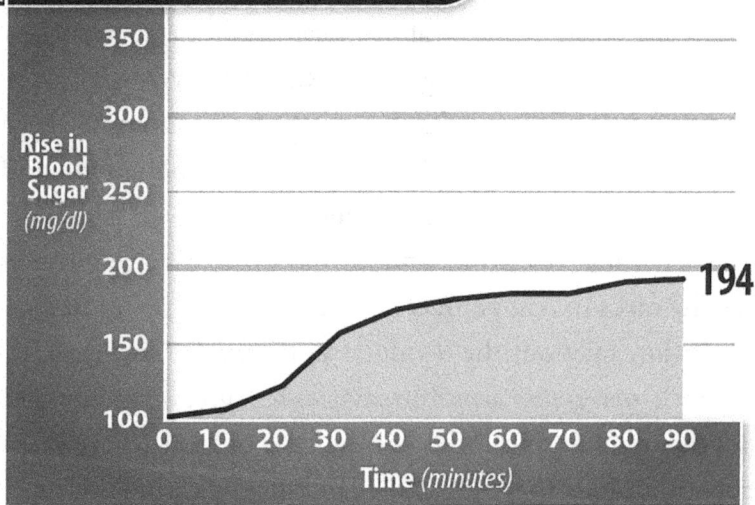

Rise in Blood Sugar (mg/dl)

350
300
250
200
150
100

0 10 20 30 40 50 60 70 80 90

194

Time (minutes)

Total Calories – 94

81 **Voskos Greek Yogurt Plain Original**

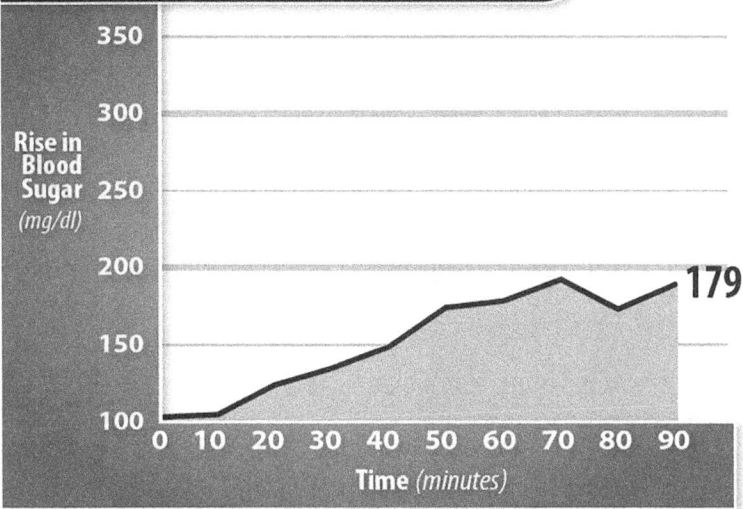

Rise in Blood Sugar *(mg/dl)*

Time *(minutes)*

179

Total Calories –79

82 **Voskos Greek Yogurt (Plain Non-fat)**

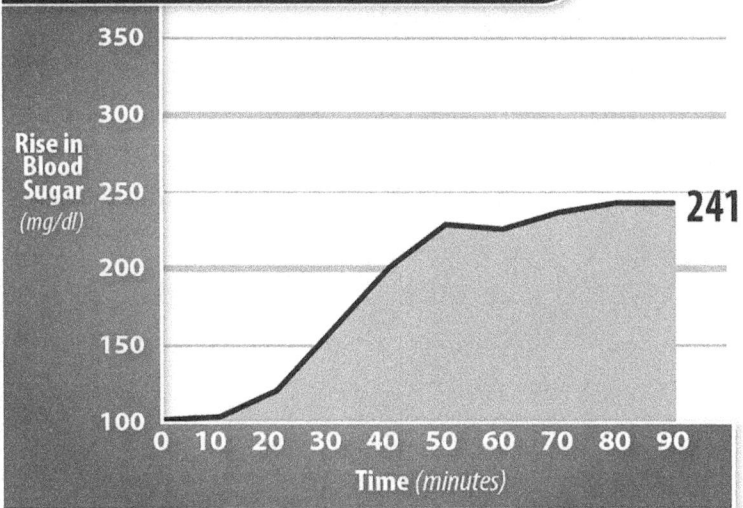

Rise in Blood Sugar *(mg/dl)*

Time *(minutes)*

241

Total Calories – 141

Chapter 6

The Type 2 Lifeline
Friends and Foes

Protein and Vegetable Carbs—Your Friends
Fat and Fruit Carbs—Your *Conditional* Friends
Starchy Carbs and Sweet Carbs—Your Foes

Now that you've had a chance to study the graphs, let's review the key points of the *Type 2 Lifeline Diet*™ that you need to lock in your mind.

Eliminate Sweet Carbohydrates—
Except for Very Special Occasions. *They Are Your Foes.*
We now know this category of foods enters your bloodstream very quickly and causes very large and fast increases in blood sugar and therefore weight. These sweet carbohydrates will show up on my blood sugar tests in two or three minutes.

The simple sugars with no fat mixed in are the quickest to enter the bloodstream and you now know that is bad. Sugared soft drinks, Skittles, jelly beans, and other candies that are simple sugars fall into this category. Baked desserts such as cakes and pies usually have some fat in them, as do chocolate candy bars and ice cream. As you now know, fat enters your bloodstream more slowly, so when fat mixes with sweet carbohydrates in your stomach, the combination is a little slower to enter your bloodstream than sweet carbohydrates by themselves. However, the fat, hitching a ride with the sweets, results in a big rise in blood sugar and a major contribution to weight.

Dramatically Minimize Starchy Carbohydrates.
They Are Your Foes.

You've seen from the graphs that this is also a category of carbohydrates that raises your blood sugar very quickly and results in an increase about as great as that of sweet carbs.

Although most people realize that sweets are big contributors to weight gain and to Type 2 diabetes, very few realize how much starchy carbs contribute to our national obesity and to our Type 2 diabetes epidemic. Starchy carbs may be even bigger contributors to our overweight problem because people in general eat a larger volume of starchy carbs than of sweets.

The best step you can take to lower your blood sugars and reduce your weight is to dramatically minimize your consumption of starchy and sweet carbohydrates.

In Dr. William Davis's excellent book, Wheat Belly (Rodale, 2011), Dr. Davis came to conclusions very similar to the conclusions I've come to. He first introduces the problem with what I call starchy carbs with the following headline on the back cover of his book, "DID YOU KNOW THAT EATING TWO SLICES OF WHOLE WHEAT BREAD CAN INCREASE BLOOD SUGAR MORE THAN TWO TABLESPOONS OF PURE SUGAR CAN?"

Early in his book he describes what he calls "wheat belly". "A wheat belly represents the accumulation of fat that results from years of consuming goods that trigger insulin, the hormone of fat storage. While some people store fat in their buttocks and thighs, most people collect ungainly fat around the middle."

Dr. Davis also talks about the lethargy and drowsiness that results from eating wheat-based foods for breakfast instead of protein and fat. He states, "I couldn't help but notice that on the days when I'd eat toast, waffles, or bagels for breakfast, I'd stumble through several hours of sleepiness and lethargy. But eat a three-egg omelet with cheese and I feel fine."

In his book, he also refers to the success that he has had with his patients who replaced wheat-based foods with other, healthier whole foods, "After three months, my patients returned to have more blood work done. As I had anticipated, with only rare exceptions, blood sugar (glucose) had indeed often dropped from diabetic range (126 mg/dl or greater) to normal. Yes, diabetics became nondiabetics. That's right: Diabetes in many cases can be cured—not simply managed—by removal of carbohydrates, especially wheat from the diet. Many of my patients lost twenty, thirty, even forty pounds."

Two items in that quote deserve a response. First, when he talks about diabetics becoming nondiabetics, I'm sure he is referring to Type 2 diabetics. Second, I don't advocate the removal of all carbohydrates from a diet. I advocate dramatically limiting sweet carbohydrates and starchy carbohydrates; protein, fat, and vegetable carbohydrates don't need to be limited at all and fruit carbohydrates just need to be slightly limited.

Eat Fruit Carbs. *Fruit Is Your Conditional Friend*
Fruit carbs vary quite a bit, but the graphs should have helped you understand their general impact. The basic message regarding fruit carbohydrates is that they will raise blood sugar a little more than veggie carbs and protein but way less than sweet or starchy carbs. Fruits include many vitamins and water-soluble fibers that are very important to general good health. Including fruits as part of your eating lifestyle is important; However, in my experience fruits such as pineapples, peaches, bananas, and strawberries will raise blood sugar fairly fast and need to be eaten in moderation in order to maintain lower blood sugars and lose weight.

Fruit juices are a different story. They are problematic in causing very fast and very big weight gains.

In many cases a large glass of apple juice, orange juice, or pineapple juice for breakfast will raise your blood sugar more and put on more weight than all the rest of your breakfast combined and it gets into your bloodstream much faster than you can use it, so it gets stored in and around your body.

An Associated Press article from the December 11, 2011 edition of the *Honolulu Star Advertiser* substantiates what I learned from my testing.

Apple juice is far from nutritious. Nutrition experts say apple juice's real danger is to waistlines and children's teeth. Apple juice has few natural nutrients, lots of calories, and in some cases, more sugar than soda. It trains a child to like very sweet things, displaces better beverages and foods, and adds to the obesity problem.

Freely Eat Veggie Carbohydrates. *They Are Your Friends*

As you learned from the graphs, vegetable carbs are an excellent group of foods for lowering blood sugar and losing weight. Not only do these foods have lots of nutrients but they also enter your bloodstream more slowly than the previous three categories. This means that you can burn the calories from these carbohydrates before they get stored as glycogen in your liver or as fat around your body. These are the foods your mom told you to eat. She was right. They include most vegetables with the exception of the starchy ones I mentioned earlier—corn and potatoes.

"Eat Produce, Live Longer" was the headline of a March 17, 2017 story in *The Week* magazine. The story went on to explain.

> *After analyzing 95 studies on diet and well-being,*
> *researchers from the Imperial College London have*
> *concluded that we should be aiming to eat 10 portions*

*of fruit and vegetables a day, rather than the five
portions recommended by the World Health
Organization. They found that the daily consumption
of 28 ounces of fresh produce was associated with a
33 percent reduced risk of stroke, a 13 percent drop
in cancer risk, and a 33 percent lower risk for
premature death.*

Freely Eat Proteins. *They Are Your Friends Too*

Proteins have gone in and out of favor many times in the past 60 years. From my experience over the past 35 years of blood sugar testing, I've made protein a very significant part of my diet to keep my blood sugars in control and weight down. Protein has very little effect on blood sugar and a very noticeably positive effect on my muscle growth when I match protein with strength training.

As you could tell from the graphs, protein will cause neither a quick nor a significant rise in blood sugar. Consequently, I freely eat large quantities of protein with a barely measurable effect on my blood sugar. Here's a review of protein that you can eat often and freely without weight gain: salmon, halibut, cod, trout, shrimp, scallops, chicken and turkey (with skin but without breading), Cornish game hen, beef, ham, and pork.

My core protein food is wild Alaska salmon. I eat it two or three times a week in the summer and maybe once a week in the winter. It's an almost perfect food. With minimal impact on my blood sugar, it's absorbed slowly so the small amount of glucose it creates is burned as fast as it goes into the bloodstream and doesn't get stored as fat. Salmon is not only very high in protein but also high in omega-3 fatty acids (which all my reading indicates is a good fat). Salmon is also a good source of vitamin D. All that and it tastes great too. Just don't overcook it.

Eat Fat. It Stabilizes Your Blood Sugar, Does Not Contribute to Weight Increases, and Many Researchers are Now Promoting Fat as a Healthy Part of a Diet.
Fat is Your Friend but Under Certain Conditions

I spend a lot more time talking about fats in this book than about any other of the food groups because my personal experiences and conclusions are significantly different from what our Government through the Department of Agriculture has told us for so many years and because it will take a lot of convincing and repetition to persuade Americans of the valuable role of dietary fat in lowering blood sugar and losing weight.

The impact of fats has been the biggest surprise to me over my years of testing—maybe revelation is a better word—and I think the same will hold true for you. You can see from the graphs in the previous chapter that adding butter to vegetables has almost no blood sugar impact, that bacon alone has minimal impact, that eggs with the yolk have almost no blood sugar impact.

I probably add more butter to my foods than 90 percent of Americans, and have for 30 years, but I eat very few baked desserts so I don't get all the butter that is combined with starchy and sweet carbs in those foods. Because most of my butter is used on vegetable carbs, my blood profile and cholesterol ratios are great. In the words of Dr. John Mues, a friend of mine and a very fit and athletic 60-year-old, "Fat is your friend."

I agree with John except I'd call fat a "conditional friend." Fat is your friend if you eat it with protein, with vegetables, or with salads. But if you eat a meal with a piece of fatty meat and also have potatoes, or biscuits, or rice, then the starchy carbs will create such an insulin demand that much of the fat will flow into the fat storage cells along with the starchy carbs.

The second reason I call fat a conditional friend is if you've had fat in your meal and you follow that meal with dessert, the fat you've eaten prior to dessert will flow along with the sweet carbs into your fat storage cells.

Here are some examples of foods that have a significant amount of natural "fats": butter, eggs (with the yolk), pork, sausage, bacon, prime rib, most steaks (especially rib eye), hamburger, bratwurst, mutton, and veal (which I don't eat because of the bad treatment of calves).

How Does the Beef Industry Make Cows
as Fat as Possible as Fast as Possible?

As I said in the lead-in to this section, fats are not the villains they are made out to be. For years we've read over and over about losing weight with low-fat diets. We've read about low-fat this and low-fat that. Who argued? It seemed so reasonable. If you don't want to be fat then don't eat fat. Simple, right? No ... wrong!

Think about this for a minute—if eating fat makes people fat, one would think it would hold true for animals too. After all, enough similarities exist between mice and humans that mice are continually being tested by scientists to see how humans might react to the same food, medications, or environmental situations.

The beef industry has an incentive to make its product as fat as possible as fast as possible. Do they feed their cows fat? No!

Over the last 80 years in America, the beef industry has learned how to make cows *as fat as possible as fast as possible.* How do they do it? They grow their cattle in feedlots on a diet of feed consisting primarily of corn and grains ... and remember I said corn was one of the two vegetables that acts like starchy carbs. I'd call this feed stock, *"starchy carbohydrates for cows."*

How often have you heard or read the term "pure corn-fed beef?" Corn- and grain-dominated feed makes cows fat quickly and gives beef a juicier, fattier texture—and likely a better taste. This is great for the beef industry and for all of us who enjoy a tasty, juicy steak; but is this what you want for yourself—*to get as fat as possible as fast as possible?*

The next time you're getting ready to eat a nice rib-eye steak remind yourself that the cow that nicely marbled steak came from ate not one ounce of fat.

What Some Others Say About This Approach

The best-known advocate for a general low-carbohydrate diet is Dr. Robert Atkins, who in 2002 wrote Dr. Atkins New Diet Revolution. Some of his conclusions were different from mine. He didn't break down carbohydrates into the categories that I believe are so important to weight loss and Type 2 diabetes reversal.

I recently saw a clip from an interview Dr. Atkins had many years ago with Barbara Walters. In this interview she said to him, "Are you telling me that I can eat as much fat as I want and won't gain weight?" He simply and emphatically said, "Yes, if you don't eat that fat with carbohydrates." That means—according to Dr. Atkins— fat is a good weight loss food only if you eat it solely with protein. That is a very limiting use of butter, for example.

My Research and Conclusions Are Somewhat Different

My conclusions are just slightly different but very important. Fat is a good weight loss tool when eaten with protein *and veggie carbs* in a meal. You can put all the butter you want on the vegetables— except for corn and potatoes—and it will contribute almost nothing to blood sugar or weight gain.

That is, in fact, a very significant difference because it shows that you can eat vegetable carbohydrates with butter or other fat and it will have very little impact on your blood sugar or weight. But if you eat butter, for example, with bread, rice, spaghetti, corn, or potatoes, or if you follow a meal with a dessert (sweet carbs) then that butter will contribute significantly to weight gain.

You will find that by putting butter liberally on vegetables as well as crab, lobster, salmon, halibut, cod, pollock, shrimp, and other seafood, you will eat more vegetables and more fish—all great contributors to weight control and good health.

Doctor Eric Westman, Director of the Duke University Lifestyle Medicine Clinic

Dr. Eric Westman, director of the Duke Lifestyle Medicine Clinic and one of the authors of *A New Atkins for a New You*, has been studying low-carbohydrate diets for 12 years and says, "...when it comes to protein and fat, eat as much as you want. You don't have to use portion control. Your hunger will go down when you start eating this way—all you have to do is stop eating when you're full." He also says, "Say good-bye to pasta, rice, bread, and corn" among other weight contributors. My testing generally confirms what Dr. Westman is saying.

Gary Taubes's Book, *Why We Get Fat—And What to Do About It.*

In an article by Lisa Davis in the February 11, 2011 issue of *Reader's Digest*, she writes about Gary Taubes's new book, *Why We Get Fat—And What to Do About It*. Taubes is an award-winning science journalist.

Davis writes,

> *If obesity researchers are so smart, why are we so large?*
> *After all, public health authorities have been*
> *hammering home a very simple message for the past 40*
> *years. If you don't want to be fat, cut the fat from your*
> *diet. And in those years, obesity rates have gone from*
> *13 percent to 22 percent to—in the last national*
> *survey—33 percent.*

Taubes thinks he know why: Obesity experts have gotten things just about completely backward. If you look carefully at the research, he says, fat isn't the enemy; easily digested carbohydrates are. The very foods that we've been sold as diet staples—fat-free yogurt, plain baked potatoes—hold the butter—and plain pasta—hold the olive oil, sauce, and cheese— actually reset our physiology to make us pack on the pounds. And the foods that we've been told to shun— steak, burgers, cheese, even the sour cream so carefully scraped from that potato—can help us finally lose the weight and keep our hearts healthy.

Taubes continues with his message under the heading "High Fat Is Better for Your Heart." Regarding the low-carb, high-fat diet he says, "Your HDL [the good cholesterol] goes up, which is the most meaningful number in terms of heart health. Not only does your cholesterol profile get better, your insulin goes down, your insulin resistance goes away, and your blood pressure goes down."

He continues, *"The low-fat diet that people have been eating in hopes of protecting their heart is actually bad for their heart."*

He argues that diets high in carbohydrates are one of the fundamental reasons that we now have obesity and diabetes epidemics. I would more specifically say that it's diets high in starchy carbohydrates and sweet carbohydrates that have been one of the biggest causes of our Type 2 diabetes epidemic.

In 2007, Taubes published *Good Calories, Bad Calories: Challenging the Conventional Wisdom on Diet, Weight Control and Disease,* a book that led the New York Times to assert that "Gary Taubes is a brave and bold science journalist" who shows that "much of what is believed about nutrition and health is based on the flimsiest evidence."

Taubes's message: Political pressure and sloppy science over the last 50 years have skewed research to make it seem that dietary fat and cholesterol are the main causes of obesity and heart disease, but there are, in fact, few or no objective data to support that hypothesis.

A more careful look (Taubes researched his book for five years; its 450 pages include 60 pages of footnotes) reveals that the real obesity-epidemic drivers are increased consumption of refined carbohydrates, mainly sugar and white flour.

Bottom line: "Carbohydrate is driving insulin and is driving fat deposition." When it comes to accumulating fat, carbohydrates are indeed "bad calories," as they are the only ones that boost insulin and make fat accumulation possible.

My 60,000 blood tests show that the villains are sweet and starchy carbs—not vegetable carbs or most fruit carbs.

What's the scientific weight-loss solution? Taubes asserted that since the fewer carbohydrates we eat, the leaner we will be, our diets should emphasize meat, fish, fowl, cheese, butter, eggs, and non-starchy vegetables.

Conversely, we should reduce, or preferably eliminate, bread and other baked goods, potatoes, yams, rice, pasta, cereal grains, corn, sugar (both sucrose and high-fructose corn syrup), ice cream, candy, soft drinks, fruit juices, bananas and other tropical fruits, and beer. Excluding carbohydrates from the diet, he said, derails the insulin peak/dip roller coaster, so one is never voraciously hungry, making weight loss and healthy-weight maintenance easy.

According to Taubes and supported by my testing, "When you eat this way, the fat just melts off."

"Sugar Tied to Fatal Heart Woes"

On February 5, 2014, the *Anchorage Daily News* ran an Associated Press Article by Lindsey Tanner. The headline was **"Sugar tied to fatal heart woes."**

The article said the American Centers for Disease Control and Prevention studied over 30,000 American adults with an average age of 44. Lead author Quanhe Yang called the results sobering and said it's the first nationally representative study to examine the issue.

The article stated, "'Scientists aren't certain exactly how sugar may contribute to deadly heart problems, but it has been shown to increase blood pressure and levels of unhealthy cholesterol and triglycerides; and also may increase signs of inflammation linked with heart disease,' said Rachel Johnson, head of the American Heart Association's nutrition committee and a University of Vermont nutrition professor."

AUTHOR'S NOTE:

I think within a few years, this type of research will also identify starchy carbs as contributors to those same heart problems, elevated cholesterol, and triglycerides caused by sugars. This is just one more bit of support for my argument that elevated glucose is a major contributor to these problems. It's not fat—unless of course the fat is accompanied in your meals by sweet or starchy carbs.

A Good Reference Book on Diabetes

One of the best books I've found on blood sugar control and health is DIABETES SOLUTION by Richard K. Bernstein, MD. It's very clearly and persuasively written by a doctor who has lived with Type 1 diabetes for "65 years and counting."

Dr. Bernstein uses the words "in theory" when he talks about acquiring more body fat from a fat-free dessert than from a "steak nicely marbled with fat." My graphs showed you that it's not just "in theory." It's reality.

The Evolution of Opinions on Fat

Here's a very visual illustration of the evolution of opinions on the role of fat in a healthy diet.

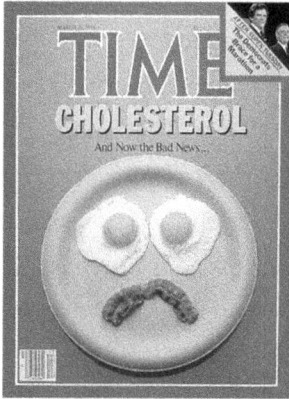

TIME Magazine
March 1994

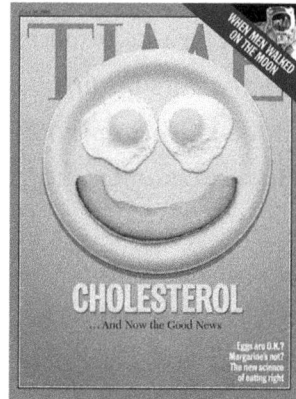

TIME Magazine
July 1999

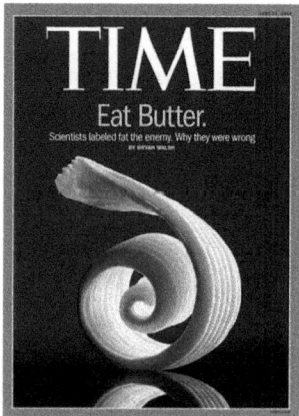

TIME Magazine
June 2014*

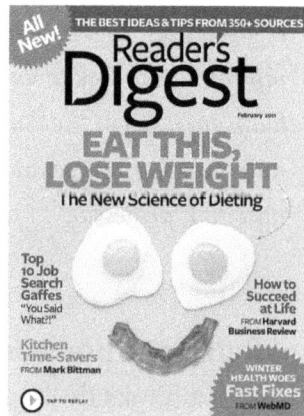

Reader's Digest
February 2011

---

* On June 23, 2014, *Time Magazine's* cover headlined the words "Eat Butter." The subhead declared "Scientists labeled fat the enemy. Why they were wrong."

Conclusion

First, remember my previous explanation that the simplest defini-tion of carbs is this: *If a food is not a protein or a fat, then it's a carb*. You now know that *sweets* are carbs, *starchy foods* are carbs, *fruits* are carbs, and *vegetables* are carbs.

What I've heard from so many people as I talk to them about Type 2 diabetes is something like, "I read that I shouldn't eat carbs" or, "My doctor said I should cut back on carbs." Does that mean eat less broccoli, fewer apples, or cut out cauliflower? No!

To really understand what you should eat and what you shouldn't eat, you must understand that carbs should not be universally con-demned or universally praised. Review the graphs, you'll see that veggie carbs along with protein are a perfect food to load up on and add all the butter you want. Fruit carbs are a little more likely to raise blood sugar but on balance are still good.

To successfully reverse Type 2 diabetes and lose weight, you must dramatically reduce starchy carbs and eliminate—or very nearly eliminate—sweet carbs.

Getting Started on Your Type 2 Diabetes Lifeline Diet

Now that you know what to eat, you just need to know how to get started.

For Type 2 diabetics, embracing this advice will eliminate your symptoms of diabetes. Some may call that curing your Type 2 dia-betes, others may call it eliminating the symptoms and avoiding the complications of diabetes. Whatever you call it, you will feel better, look better, be slimmer, and be healthier.

Apply my advice and you'll be on your way to a longer, healthier life.

The next chapter will get you started on lowering your blood sugars and reversing Type 2 diabetes on either a one-month or two-month schedule—your choice.

Chapter 7

Getting Started on Your Diabetes Lifeline™ Diet

Easy Changes for a two-month schedule to reverse Type 2 diabetes & Harder Changes to reverse Type 2 diabetes in one month.

Eating Lifestyle Changes—Comparing Degrees of Difficulty to Degrees of Benefit

You'll see in this chapter that some of the lifestyle changes are very easy, some are slightly harder, and some are very hard. You'll also find that the degrees of benefit vary. Some changes in your diet will make a small difference in your blood sugars, weight, and health in the short run but will still be significant in the long run. Other changes will have a bigger benefit right away and will be even more significant over the months and years. And some changes will have a dramatic impact very quickly and will reverse Type 2 diabetes in just one month and be life-changing over the years.

You'll stumble or falter a bit along the way but the changes will be worth it. Remember, each of these changes is part of the whole package of lifestyle changes that together will give you a healthier life. You don't have to embrace and adopt them all but the more of them you do the healthier you'll be. Nor do you have to be perfect in your eating lifestyle—only good.

Explaining the Lifeline Grid

I struggled for a long time with how to present these actions by ease or difficulty of the action and significance of the benefit. Should I assign a number, sort of like degree of difficulty in diving or gymnastics? That didn't work because it implied a degree of specificity that was not defensible. The same applied to the degree of benefit. How do you assign a valid numeric value to the different changes I've recommended? Finally, I came up with the idea of a Diabetes Lifeline Grid. Along the horizontal axis (X axis) is the degree of difficulty and along the vertical axis (Y axis) is the degree of benefit.

As you look at the Diabetes Lifeline Grid, you'll see that the action in the lower left-hand quadrant of the grid is easy and has modest benefit. Those actions that are higher in that quadrant are more beneficial and those that are farther right are slightly more difficult.

Diabetes Lifeline Grid

Going clockwise from the lower left to the upper left-hand quadrant, you'll find those actions that are still easy and have great benefit in both the short and long term. Focus on these actions immediately. As in all quadrants, the higher they are the greater the benefit and the farther right the higher the difficulty. In the upper right quadrant are the actions that will be harder but will have great short- and long-term benefits. These are the changes that you'll have to work at, but they will be life-changing. Finally, in the lower right-hand quadrant would be changes that are hard and will have little benefit. I haven't even discussed anything that conceivably might fit in that quadrant and would have no reason to do so.

Conclusion

Review the changes listed and then review the location of each change on the lifestyle graph. After you've considered the benefit

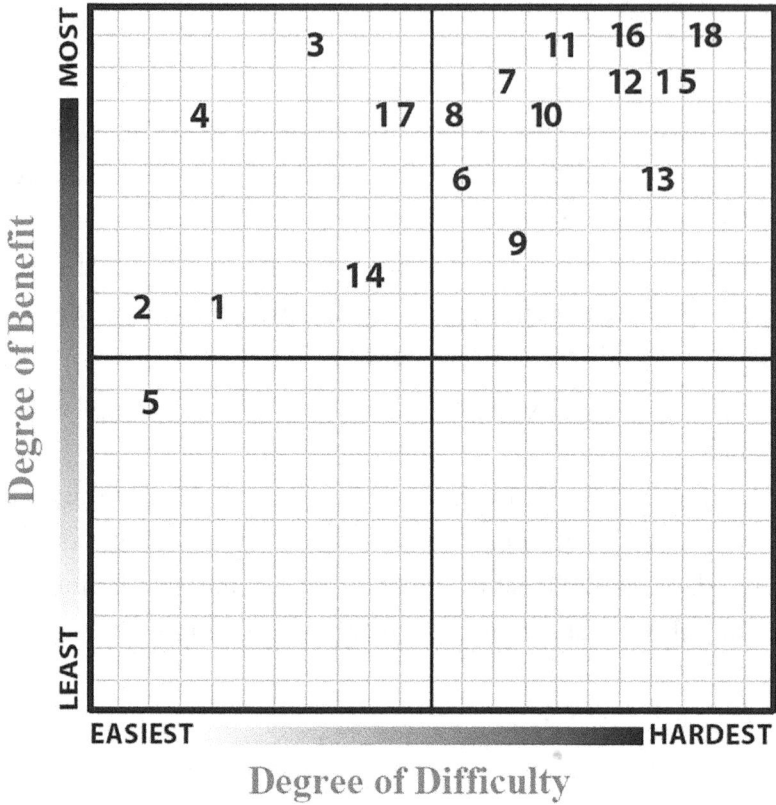

and the ease or difficulty of those changes, decide which you want to include in your new eating lifestyle.

If you're serious about reversing Type 2 diabetes quickly and losing weight fast, take note of the eating actions in bold type. Your blood sugars will drop and weight loss will start right away and will continue. When you reach your ideal weight, don't go back to your old way of eating—instead, just slide back to some of the nonbolded actions.

Breakfast

1. Reduce starchy carbs in your breakfast.

2. Eat egg-white omelets if you have any starchy carbs at all.

3. **Eliminate starchy carbs from your breakfast—no cereal, no toast or muffins, no potatoes.**

4. **Add more protein and vegetables to your breakfast—whole eggs and butter are okay if you eat no sweet or starchy carbs.**

5. **Dilute your breakfast juices.**

Lunch

6. Reduce starchy carbs in your lunches and eat more protein and vegetables.

7. **Eliminate starchy carbs at lunch and eat only protein, fat, vegetables, and maybe a small amount of fruit for lunch—butter and salad dressing are okay.**

8. Eliminate desserts at lunch.

Dinner

9. **Eat dinner earlier.**

10. Eat more protein and vegetables and fewer starchy carbs for dinner.

11. **Eat only protein, vegetables, and a small portion of fruit for dinner** (butter and salad dressings are okay if you eat at least three hours before going to sleep).

12. **Reduce portion size for dinner at home and in restaurants.**

13. Share an entree with your dinner partner at restaurants.

14. Order an appetizer—or maybe two— in place of dinner at restaurants.

15. Ask for half of your meal to be put in a to-go box before you get it.

After-Dinner Snacks

16. **Eliminate eating desserts as a regular habit—special occasions are okay.**

17. Improve and/or reduce your after-dinner snacks.

18. **Eliminate your after-dinner snacks.**

AUTHOR'S NOTE:
If you're really serious about lowering blood sugar and losing weight fast, take note of the eating actions I put in bold type.

Chapter 8

Developing Your Type 2 Lifeline Diet Patterns

So far you learned a lot about what foods do lower your blood sugars, lighten the workload of your pancreas, and cause weight loss, and what foods *do not*; now you need tips on how to apply that information and convert what you've learned to a new eating lifestyle that will be easy to maintain.

Reversing or avoiding Type 2 diabetes, losing weight, and becoming healthier is about changing lifestyles. It's about setting new patterns of eating and then making those patterns habits.

Once you start the eating patterns of the *Diabetes Lifeline Diet*™, you will start lowering your blood sugars and losing weight right away. When you continue those patterns, you will continue lowering your blood sugars and losing weight.

At first, you'll have to think about it every day. It will be easier now that you know which foods to eat and which to avoid, but it will take some discipline to continue losing weight. But when you follow these patterns for a couple of months, the patterns will become habits; then you won't even have to think about it.

When you wake up in the morning, you don't look at a note that says, "Brush your teeth and wash your face." You don't need to think about getting a cup of coffee, getting the newspaper from your porch or opening the news up on your tablet, or having your normal breakfast. You just do it. And you certainly don't need a note that says, "Say good morning," to your husband, wife, or partner. You've established certain patterns and they've just become habits.

Here you'll find tips to change your eating patterns, lower your blood sugars, and help you start losing weight. You need to make those patterns into eating lifestyle habits that will keep your blood sugars normal and keep weight off for the rest of your life.

By way of warning, once you've reached your desired weight, don't go back to your old eating lifestyle; just increase the portion size of the better food that you are now eating in your *Diabetes Lifeline Diet™*.

Let's start with breakfast.

Breakfast

1. Be Sure to Dilute (or avoid) Fruit Juices

You saw in chapter 5 how fast and how much orange juice and apple juice raise blood sugar and add to weight.

The pattern you need to start here is to *avoid or dilute juice*. Some people, as I do, have juice only periodically in the morning but many of you may drink juice at different times throughout the day thinking that it's the healthy thing to do. *It's not.*

The impact on your blood sugar and weight counteracts the positive benefit you may get. Though I didn't include pineapple juice in the graphs, it's similar to orange and apple juice in its impact.

The way to get some benefit from the vitamins that are present in juices is to dilute your juices before you drink them. In the morning, I fill about ¼ of a juice glass with the juice and fill the rest with water. You'll be surprised how easy it is to get used to diluted juices. It won't take long before full-strength orange juice feels very thick and very sugary.

The best juice for keeping blood sugar and weight down is V-8 juice. You can choose to dilute it but that's not necessary. I dilute V-8 juice by using a full-size 8-ounce glass—not a juice glass— and putting about ½ glass of V-8 juice in it and filling the rest with water or sparkling water. It's a very refreshing drink that you will soon become accustomed to.

An Example of Losing Over 20 Pounds
Solely by Cutting Back on Orange Juice

The benefit you reap from this change will depend on how much juice you currently drink. If you're a big juice drinker, the benefit will be great. A good example of a huge benefit comes via Barbara Mee, a longtime friend and former special assistant to the late Senator Ted Stevens. Barbara had heard me speak about diabetes. Among the tips I suggested to lower blood sugar and lose weight was to dilute or eliminate certain juices.

Barbara's husband, Vince, worked in street maintenance for the Municipality of Anchorage. His work at that time involved driving snowplows in the winter and driving trucks the rest of the year. Vince was overweight at the time and thinking he was being very conscientious about his health, he started his day with a big 20-ounce mug of orange juice in his plow.

Soon after Barbara told him about my orange juice suggestion, Vince—coincidentally—had a doctor's appointment. He told the doctor about my advice and the doctor strongly agreed. According to Vince, the doctor told him he needed to lose weight and the first thing he should do was "get off that orange juice." "That's like mainlining sugar," Vince quoted his doctor as saying. Vince immediately quit drinking it on the job and cut way back to just a little diluted orange juice for breakfast. Barbara said within months Vince had lost

"20 to 25 pounds solely by cutting back on the huge amount of orange juice he drank."

Now both Barbara and Vince are enjoying a well-deserved and active retirement in Florida. They're playing golf together five or six days a week. Vince has never regained the weight he lost after cutting way back on orange juice.

2. Eliminate or Dramatically Reduce Toast, Muffins, and Bagels for Breakfast

For so many years, many health-conscious people thought eating some toast, a bagel with cream cheese or a muffin was a decent, healthy breakfast. *Not so.* In terms of weight gain let's look at these choices.

Toast and English Muffins

If you can't eliminate them, at least eat very small portions, like half of a piece of toast or a quarter of a muffin. But if you eat two pieces of toast that's quadruple the starchy carbs. And if you add jelly or jam that's another 30 calories of sweet carbs that will get into your bloodstream so fast that unless you run to work, you won't burn it before it will get stored in the liver as glycogen and then later on your stomach, legs, or hips as fat.

Bagels

Bagels are big. Bagels are starchy. Bagels will send your blood sugar through the roof and make you fat. They will be converted to glucose and enter your bloodstream as glucose faster than you can burn that glucose. Eliminate bagels from your breakfast.

Cinnamon and Sugar vs. Jam or Jelly

If you must have a piece of toast in the morning, do yourself a favor and put a mixture of sugar and cinnamon on it instead of jam or jelly. What— sugar? Yes, cinnamon and sugar. Years ago when I still ate toast for breakfast, I had a feeling that jelly on my toast had a bigger impact on my blood sugar than cinnamon and sugar. I started experimenting with my blood testing and found out it was true.

As an experiment, I put the same amount of cinnamon and sugar that I put on my toast into a teaspoon. It turned about to be ½ teaspoon. Figuring the sugar was about 50 percent of the mixture, I was putting about ¼ teaspoon of sugar on my toast. At 17 calories per teaspoon of sugar I was adding a little more than 4 calories to my toast; compare that to 32 to 36 calories that jelly added. Some would say it's not a big deal; it only saves about 30 calories a day.

I'd say look at it this way: that simple, small daily action if done daily, would save 210 calories a week, which is the number of calories in one Hershey bar. That means putting jelly or jam on your toast every morning instead of cinnamon and sugar is equivalent to adding 52 Hershey bars a year to your eating pattern. This is such a good illustration of how making a little change in a daily habit can add up to a meaningful weight loss in a year. Of course, it's much better if you just don't eat toast at all.

3. Eliminate Cereal from Your Breakfast Pattern

Remember when we were kids? We'd wake up and pour ourselves as much cereal as would fit in the bowl, put lots of sugar on it, maybe a banana, and then go out and play for three or four hours. If you're going out after breakfast to play for three or four hours, go ahead and load up on cereal. But if you're not, you must cut back—or eliminate cereal. Look at the graphs one more time and note the impact of cereal on your blood sugar and your weight.

It's the starchy carbohydrate issue. Unless you're going to be very active after breakfast, the cereal will be stored faster than you will burn it and it will trigger storage of the glucose in your blood. You're much better off cutting out cereal and eating eggs, some vegetable, and some breakfast meat—if you wish—for your breakfast. The protein and fat in the egg and meat option will go very slowly into your bloodstream and allow you to burn the small amount of glucose that protein and fat create before it ever gets stored.

4. Do Not Eat Sweet Carbohydrates for Breakfast

I'm sure most of you don't do that but if you do eat doughnuts or sweet rolls for breakfast, *stop* for the sake of your blood sugar control, your weight, and your health. Review the charts in chapter 5 and see how much a single medium Cherry Danish or a donut will raise blood sugar in just 90 minutes.

5. Eat More Protein for Breakfast

If you're cutting back on the above, then what *should* you eat for breakfast? The answer is more *protein and vegetables*. Don't worry about the fat that comes along with it. The breakfast that I recommend starts with eggs. My preference for breakfast is two or three eggs boiled, fried, scrambled, or poached—without toast. I will almost always add a vegetable—most often cauliflower—to my breakfast and put butter on the vegetable.

Add bacon freely to your breakfast. As long as you have no starchy carbs or sweets, the bacon will have only a miniscule impact on your blood sugar and weight.

Now when should you eat an egg-white omelet and when should you eat a whole-egg omelet? I'll eat an egg-white omelet if I'm going to do a strength workout because an egg-white omelet usually has the whites of six or seven eggs—that means 42 to 49 grams of protein, whereas a whole-egg omelet usually consists of three complete eggs, and has only 21 grams of protein. More protein will help you improve the ration of muscle to fat whether you're a man or a woman.

When I say that fat will not significantly add to your blood sugar or weight, that's true as long as you don't eat starchy or sweet carbs with the meal. Here's more specific timing. *Based on my blood sugar testing, I've learned that in order to keep your blood low after eating fat, you should not eat starchy or sweet carbs one hour before a meal with fat in it, during a meal with fat in it, or three hours after the meal with fat in it.*

6. Eat Vegetables for Breakfast

Who eats vegetables for breakfast? The truth is not many Americans do unless they are making a veggie omelet or a fritata. But we're missing out on a great health addition for our first meal of the day.

I stopped eating toast and started eating tomato slices for breakfast years ago. Then I moved into different vegetables. Now I almost always have a healthy portion of either asparagus, broccoli, or cauliflower, each with melted butter. Once I started that habit I started losing weight quickly even though that wasn't necessarily my goal.

Like the fat in bacon and eggs, the butter fat will have little impact on your blood sugar. Switching away from starchy carbs for breakfast and to protein and vegetables with or without butter is one of the easiest and most effective ways to reduce blood sugar and lose weight. I choose to use butter with my vegetables because vegetables taste so much better with butter. My daily consumption of vegetables has gone up and my blood sugar and weight have gone down.

In Summary, Follow This Lifeline Pattern for Breakfast

Dilute your juices.

Eliminate *starchy carbohydrates* such as bread, muffins, cereal, and potatoes.

Eat more *protein* and *fat*.

Do not eat sweet rolls, donuts, or any other *sweet carbohydrates* for breakfast.

Start adding a *vegetable or vegetables* to your breakfast.

If you start that breakfast eating pattern you will be well on your way to lowering your blood sugar and easing the strain on your pancreas. In addition, you will start losing weight because the glucose from those foods will go very slowly into your bloodstream and you'll have three or more hours to burn that glucose before it's stored around your body in all the places you don't want it stored: mostly stomach for men, and legs and hips for women.

That slow entry into your bloodstream also results in a much more diminished sense of hunger at lunch than you would have if you had eaten cereal, bagels, or any other starchy carbs. You will be less likely to eat a big lunch.

To keep your blood low after eating fat, you should not eat starchy or sweet carbs one hour before a meal with fat in it, during a meal with fat in it, or three hours after the meal with fat in it.

But breakfast is just one part of the eating equation. The other three parts are lunch, dinner, and snacks. Next let's look at lunch.

Lunch

1. Minimize Starchy Carbs for Lunch

Once again, do everything you can to minimize starchy carbs. At lunch time, starchy carbs often enter your eating patterns in the form of bread on sandwiches, buns on burgers or hot dogs, rolls, bagels, French fries, potato chips, taco shells, tortilla chips, rice, and pasta.

A note on bread: White bread, wheat and multigrain bread all have a similar high impact on blood sugar and weight gain. If you must eat bread, then eat only very small portions. Whole grain or whole wheat are slightly better for you and have slightly less impact on blood sugar than multigrain or white bread. Still, it's better if you can eliminate bread altogether.

2. Eliminate Dessert from Lunch

Most desserts are combinations of sweet and starchy carbs such as cakes and pies or combinations of sweet and fatty carbs such as ice cream. Remember those combinations are blood-sugar-raising, weight-gaining bombshells. Do not eat dessert for lunch.

3. Eat Plenty of Protein, Fat, and Veggie Carbs for Lunch

Don't worry about holding back on protein, fat, or veggie carbs for lunch. Remember a salad consists mostly of veggie carbs and you can put dressing on the salad with near impunity as long as you don't eat any starchy carbs (including croutons) or have any sweets just before lunch, during lunch, or for three hours after lunch.

Most people already know how good vegetables are for you but I'll repeat again what most people *don't know* that's even better. Veggie carbs are so slow to enter your bloodstream as glucose that you are very likely to burn that glucose before it's ever stored.

Protein is also absorbed slowly and fat is the slowest of all foods to reach your bloodstream and fat cells. That's one of the reasons why most diabetic regimens don't even recommend counting grams of protein or fat—and they shouldn't count grams of vegetable carbohydrates. These three groups for lunch will help you eliminate snacking in the afternoon and leave you less hungry by dinnertime. Enjoy as much as you want from those three groups.

4. Fruit is Okay for Lunch

If you follow my suggestions above but do have fruit with your lunch, it will be a slightly bigger blood sugar and weight contributor than the protein, fat, and vegetables. So if you do have fruit, don't have too much. The best fruits for any meal are blueberries, blackberries, raspberries, or cantaloupe.

But if fruit is your biggest weight contributor for lunch you're going to do just fine and continue to lose weight.

By following this *Diabetes Lifeline Eating Pattern* I described for breakfast, you won't be as hungry at lunchtime and by following the pattern I described for lunch, you won't be as hungry at dinnertime. That also means you'll be less likely to snack after these meals.

I do realize that it isn't always a sense of hunger that dictates whether we snack or not. Often we snack just for something to do. I talk more about this later.

In Summary, Follow these Lifeline Steps for Lunch:

Minimize starchy carbs at lunch.

Eliminate sweet carbs (any sugars and desserts) at lunch.

Eat more protein, fat, and veggie carbs at lunch.

A limited amount of fruit is okay.

Dinner

I don't recommend eating fatty foods as freely for dinner as I do for breakfast or lunch because fat takes as long as three to four hours to get into your bloodstream. That's good for breakfast and lunch, because the fat goes in so slowly that you can burn it in your daily activity. But if you eat dinner too late, the glucose from the fatty foods will be going into your body while you're sleeping and that, of course, is not good. You burn so little glucose while you sleep that most of this glucose won't be used. It *will* be stored.

Dinner is the meal that is the biggest contributor to blood sugar elevation and weight gain in America. It's the meal that is *least* likely to have its calories burned by postmeal activity, and it's the meal most likely to have dessert associated with it.

I was eating dinner with a friend last week and he said, "Look at you. You don't even have to think about what you eat for dinner." My answer was short and quick. "That's not correct. I've been thinking about what I eat for 30 years." It's true. I rarely sit down for dinner and just "dig in." At meals, I'm always thinking about minimizing starchy carbs, sweet carbs (dessert), and at dinner I also think about minimizing fat. The key word here is *minimizing* fat, not eliminating it.

We all desire some starchy carbs at times and we're all going to have desserts periodically. But the important issue—that you're now aware of— is the huge impact that both sweet carbs and starchy carbs will have on your blood sugar and on weight gain.

Think of it this way. If the price of gasoline were to go up by two dollars a gallon tomorrow, we probably wouldn't just flat out stop driving but we would be much more cautious about how much we would drive and every time we got in our car, the impact on our pocketbook would likely be on our minds. So think about starchy carbs and sweet carbs like that. We're all going to eat them from time to time, but when you do, think about the impact on your blood glucose and weight. Just keep minimizing those blood sugar elevators until their absence ultimately becomes your habit.

If we're having a special dinner with warm, aromatic rolls being passed around the dinner table, I'm going to have one—with butter, of course, even though I know that's bad for me. If we're having company for dinner and a dessert is served, I often will have a small portion. These small enjoyments are an important part of life. I haven't given them up completely and you don't have to either. But remember—make them special, make them rare—*not part of your regular dinner routine.*

So what should you eat for dinner? The good thing about breaking down foods into the six groups instead of just three is that you'll know simply which *food groups* you can *maximize* and which *food groups* you should *minimize*. With that knowledge, lowering your blood sugars, losing weight, and keeping it off will be much easier.

1. Eat Dinner as Early as You Reasonably Can

The earlier you eat dinner, the better the opportunity to use the glucose in your bloodstream for energy rather than for storage. In the activity chapter, I'll talk about how much my insulin demand is reduced after dinner by some small activity such as walking around the yard, going out to the store, or other similar activities. More activity after dinner is, of course, better but even a small amount will make a difference as you will learn later.

2. Minimize *Starchy* Carbs For Dinner
Just Like You Do For All Other Meals.

Here's where you must be careful of the two veggie carbs that act like starchy carbs—corn and potatoes. You don't have to eliminate them, just minimize them.

Minimize or eliminate breads, rolls, rice, and pasta. In all these foods the brown versions are just slightly better than white versions. But work hard at eliminating all starchy carbs except for very special meals.

Some Fruit Is Okay

In terms of blood sugar and strain on your pancreas, fruit is somewhere in between the good groups—protein, fat, and vegetables—and the bad groups—sweet and starchy carbs. So be cautious and try to stick with berries and cantaloupe.

Go ahead and have fruit with or after dinner if you choose but don't overindulge and don't put the fruit on ice cream—sorry to tell you that.

3. Freely Eat Protein and Veggie Carbs at Dinner as Well as Fat Under Specific Conditions

Fish, poultry, meat, and veggie carbohydrates should be the core of your dinner. The skin is okay on poultry and fat is okay on meat and butter is certainly okay on fish or seafood. If you are going to have some fat for dinner you need to avoid starchy and sweet carbs in that meal and eat your dinner at least three hours before going to bed.

At home I have typical dinners of grilled, blackened, or baked Alaska salmon, cod, or halibut. Crab and shrimp are also two of my favorites. These seafoods plus pollock and lobster have almost negligible impact on blood sugar and weight.

Maybe three or four times a month I have chicken instead of fish and a few times a month I have steak. Both chicken—including the skin but not including breading—and steak are very good for keeping blood sugar low and weight down if you don't have starchy carbs in the same meal or sweet carbs for dessert.

My veggie carbs are typically broccoli, cauliflower, asparagus, green beans, and a variety of mixed salads with lettuce, vegetables, nuts, and fruit and topped with blue cheese dressing.

Protein, fat, and vegetable carbs *with butter* will not alone increase either your blood sugar or weight; but when you add starchy carbs or sweet carbs to the meal or after the meal everything changes. Your blood sugar will go up dramatically and your weight will do the same.

A significant concern about having fat for dinner is how slowly the fat makes its way into your bloodstream compared to the other food groups.

A Reminder of How Fast Different Food Groups Get Into Your Bloodstream

Sweet carbs get into your bloodstream within three to ten minutes and most often get stored as body fat before you can burn the glucose they create.

Starchy carbs get into your bloodstream in 10 to 30 minutes and unless you're exercising or very active after eating, they will also be stored as body fat.

Protein and veggie carbs go in much more slowly and that means you'll have sufficient time to burn the glucose they create before it's stored.

Fat is the slowest of all foods to enter your bloodstream. It takes from one to five hours to break down and enter the bloodstream as glucose. That's good if you eat fat for breakfast, lunch, or an early dinner because you'll have plenty of time to burn the glucose it creates before it ever has a chance to be stored as body fat. But that's bad if you eat a late dinner and go to sleep within an hour or two after eating. The fat will continue going into your bloodstream as glucose while you're sleeping and your blood sugar will continue rising for the first four of five hours you're sleeping and will *not get* burned but *will* get stored as body fat.

So remember you can eat butter on vegetables and fatty meat for dinner but an early dinner is much better than a late dinner for keeping blood sugar and weight under control. If you do eat a late dinner, you should minimize fat.

4. Reduce Portion Sizes for Dinner

Portion size for dinner is more important than portion size for breakfast and lunch. It's the meal you're least likely to burn and most likely to store as fat simply because you usually will not have as much activity after dinner as you have after breakfast or lunch.

At first, you'll find it hard to think about dinner as a small meal. When I was a child and a teenager at home my dad would finish a big dinner, typically of fried chicken, roast beef, or meat loaf with mashed potatoes and gravy, often with corn and biscuits and then lean back in his chair and declare with great satisfaction, "I feel like a million bucks." It was his way of saying he was full and, as a child of the depression, being full was good to Dad.

You may have grown up with the same messages I heard every day. "Take all you want but eat all you take." "Clean your plate." "Eat your potatoes." The intent was all positive but when you hear it over and over you cannot help but think eating a lot is good and not eating very much is bad.

If you can adopt a mindset that being full after dinner is not necessarily good, you'll be well on your way to improving your blood sugar control, losing weight, and sleeping much better.

I know this is not easy but if you can start making smaller dinners your pattern, it will eventually become your habit. You'll slip and backslide a little as you start making dinner a smaller meal. Don't say, "I failed and can't do this." Promise yourself you'll do better tomorrow.

Two suggestions for starting the habit of "dinner as a smaller meal."

1. Make a promise to yourself to eat your dinner for one month from a dessert plate. This will constantly remind you of your goal to make dinner a smaller meal. If you can do that for one month, you'll find yourself eating less and feeling better right away. When you feel you know what a smaller dinner is and when you think you can continue eating smaller even if your plate is bigger, go back to a normal dinner plate. You'll find a feeling of pride as your dinner plate actually has spaces among your helpings of food.

2. Start making a checkmark for each day you're successful in making dinner a small meal. Maybe the first week you'll be successful for only three dinners out of seven. The next week shoot for four or five days of success with your new pattern. Keep on doing that until you've succeeded all seven days in a week. Then shoot for a second consecutive week of that pattern. Once you get to four consecutive weeks, *you'll be very close to making small dinners your habit.*

You Can Do It

Eating the foods I recommend in smaller portion sizes will not only help you start losing weight and gaining control of your blood sugar right away, but more importantly, it can become a healthy eating habit that will help keep you lean and trim for the rest of your life.

I make a special point throughout these chapters of saying "typical" dinners and not "every" dinner because we all want special dinners on occasion. That's simply an important part of life. Don't give up those times. Enjoy them but even on those special times don't go overboard on starchy carbohydrates or desserts.

How About Snacking

There is a danger, however, in smaller dinner portions. The temptation to snack after dinner and before you go to bed will be even greater. How can you deal with that temptation?

5. After-Dinner Snacks

I've talked about breakfast, lunch, and dinner. Of those three meals, dinner is the meal most likely to contribute to weight gain and blood sugar problems. But right up there with dinner as a big contributor to weight gain is what's eaten after dinner—evening snacks.

Like dinner, an evening snack is a habit that is less likely to be followed by activity. When you're snacking after dinner you're contributing mightily to blood sugar increases and weight gain. After years and years of testing my blood sugar after dinner while sometimes snacking and sometimes not, here are six conclusions I've arrived at.

1. After-dinner snacks are bigger contributors to weight gain and blood sugar increases than are post-breakfast and post-lunch snacks. This may be an obvious conclusion simply because we're all more likely to burn some glucose from snacks we eat at 10 a.m. or 3 p.m. than snacks we eat at 8 or 9 p.m. Those late-evening snacks are much more likely to be stored as fat than burned.

I've never been in the habit of eating a midmorning or midafternoon snack and I don't recommend either one but they are not as impactful on weight and blood sugar as a post-dinner snack.

2. If you are going to snack after dinner, stay away from ice cream or potato chips. They will not only raise your blood sugar (and weight) because of the sweet and starchy carbs, but also,

because of their fat content they will both continue to increase your blood sugar for four or more hours after you eat them. By that time, you're likely going to be asleep and subject to the worst-case scenario of increasing blood sugar while you're burning very few calories and therefore subjecting yourself to increasing blood sugar and weight gain during the night.

3. If you feel you must snack, the best by far is a veggie selection or some protein. My favorite veggie snacks are broccoli, cauliflower, carrots and radishes with blue cheese dressing. The dressing is okay as long as you don't have any starchy carbs such as crackers with it. For protein snacks, I like smoked salmon, shrimp, or reindeer sausage.

4. A good way to improve your snacks is, "Don't buy the bad stuff." If you do buy ice cream, potato chips, candy, and similar snacks—whether you keep them visible or try to hide them from yourself—*you will eat them.* It's easier to resist them at the grocery store than to resist them in your home.

5. My next suggestion is to ask yourself when you're most likely to eat sweet or starchy snacks. I'm guessing it's when you're watching TV or in front of your computer. Before you sit down, ask yourself what else you could snack on besides sweets. As I'm writing this, I'm snacking on walnuts roasted for a salad yesterday. Even with the healthier snacks I suggested in the last paragraph, do not eat them by the handful. Eat them one at a time and take a little time in between. I've learned over the years to eat snacks less frequently and more slowly and savor each bite a little more. By doing that you will automatically be eating a little less. It's a good pattern to get into and soon you'll find it has become a habit.

6. The best plan of all is *not to snack after dinner*. If you can accomplish that you will have taken one of the biggest weight-loss and blood-sugar-lowering steps possible.

One of the best ways to avoid snacks after dinner is to be more active between dinner and bedtime. That not only decreases the likelihood of snacking but also burns glucose and lowers insulin demand.

In Summary, Follow These Diabetes Lifeline Eating Patterns for Dinner:

Eat dinner as early as you reasonably can.

Minimize *starchy* carbs just like you do for other meals.

Eliminate *sweet carbs (desserts)* after dinner.

Some fruits are okay but moderate them.

Freely eat protein and veggie carbs at dinner.

Eat fat only with early dinners and with no sweet or starchy carbs.

Reduce portion sizes for dinner.

Minimize or eliminate after-dinner snacks.

Some Tips for Eating Out

Why I Haven't Included "Breakfast Out" in this Section

Breakfast choices are typically much narrower than lunch and dinner choices. Any discussion about *eating breakfasts out* would be much the same as eating breakfast at home and therefore repetitive.

Lunch Out

Good Lunch Choices at National-Franchise Sit-Down Restaurants
As you begin lowering blood sugars and losing weight by cutting back on sweets and starchy carbs and adding protein, vegetables, and fat, here are some thoughts on restaurant options.

Here's my suggestion for a healthier lunch technique if I'm eating in franchise restaurants like Chili's, TGIF, Appleby's, Red Robin and so forth. I'll order a hamburger, a fish sandwich (not breaded), a chicken sandwich, or a turkey sandwich, or pastrami. I'll always ask if they have an alternative to French fries. If they don't, then I'll do without anything but the burger because once French fries make it to your plate, they will also make it to your mouth.

Most of the time, however, you will be able to get a vegetable alternative. It's an opportunity to have another helping of some vegetable. When you get your food, take the top off the sandwich and set it aside. Use your knife and fork to eat the meat, chicken, turkey, pastrami, or fish and the onions, tomatoes, and lettuce in the sandwich, then leave the bottom half of the sandwich on your plate. By leaving both halves of the bun behind, you've contributed greatly to lowering blood glucose and losing weight.

This, of course, also holds true for lunch at any other restaurant that serves lunch. I just used national-franchise restaurants as an example because of their standardized menus.

Fast-Food Restaurants
Like most people, I find myself at fast food restaurants once in a while. For me that's one to three times a month. For some it may be as much as seven or more times a week. Eating too often at fast food restaurants can be a problem—but not necessarily. Here are my recommendations for ways to eat fast foods that will keep your blood sugar, insulin demand, and weight down.

Arby's

Arby's has a large roast beef sandwich that I really like. Here's my pattern for eating it. I always ask for one of their plastic forks. Then I sit down, take the top half of the bun off and just eat the roast beef with Arby's horsey sauce and when I'm done I throw both halves of the bun away. That has very little impact on my blood sugar or insulin demand and I'm always amazed at how they can make roast beef so juicy.

Carl's Jr

Carl's Jr. will do all their burger choices in a low-carb format. That's one of my favorite fast-food burgers. It's simply any of their burgers wrapped in lettuce instead of a bun. That diminishes dramatically the impact it has on blood sugar, insulin demand, and weight. It's a little big so I don't always eat it all and have quit trying to eat it in my car as take-out. It can be messy. I usually sit down in the restaurant and eat it there. You get a lot of meat and you won't be hungry again until dinner.

Subway

Subway offers a lot of choices. Now that you know about veggie carbs and protein you can use that information in your selections. My pattern is to order the six-inch instead of the 12-inch sandwich then just eat one half of the bun.

Mexican Restaurants

Most Mexican foods as prepared in Mexican restaurants in America have a lot of fat, starchy carbs and some protein as primary ingredients. Generally bad combinations for Type 2 diabetics or anyone who is interested in losing weight. If you do eat in a Mexican restaurant it's better to eat there for lunch than for dinner. You'll have more time to burn off the large amount of glucose that will result.

If you can order something like fajitas, that have the protein and vegetables separated and are easily eaten without having to eat the starchy-carb wrappings, you should do that. Also cut way back on the refried beans and rice as they are very starchy and will have a big impact on your blood sugar and weight.

In general, Mexican-American food is very popular but not good for anyone with Type 2 diabetes or anyone who is pre-diabetic or borderline diabetic or trying to lose weight. It's inexpensive, fast, and tasty but be aware of the big contribution to your blood glucose and weight.

Dinner Out

Portion Size—the Biggest Problem in Most of America's Restaurants

About 15 years ago I had flown down from Alaska to visit my mom in Southern California. Instead of flying home after the visit, I decided to do something a little different and take a train, the Sunset Limited, from Los Angeles to Seattle and then fly home to Alaska from Seattle. As the train rolled north through the hills of the San Joaquin Valley, I sat down at a nicely set table in the dining car for lunch and was joined by a Dutch couple. They had been touring America by auto and were now taking the train to Seattle to catch a flight home to Holland.

They were very pleasant, congenial, and open people. Unfortunately, I've forgotten their names so I'll just call them Mr. and Mrs. Holland.

I asked them the obvious question, "What's your impression of America?" With no hesitation, Mrs. Holland blurted out, "Big." I said, "Big? Well, yes America is a big country." She said, "No, it's not just the country—it's everything. Everything's big." I knew they had talked between themselves about this because Mr. Holland continued her thought. "The mountains are big. The roads are big. The cars are big. The people are big, and the food in the restaurants is big."

Well, I'd never heard anyone call restaurant food "big" but they continued laughing and describing a litany of the large portions of food that they had been served at the last half dozen restaurants they had patronized along their journey.

In the years since that conversation, I've become more sensitive to portion sizes in restaurants. The Dutch couple was absolutely correct. The portions in restaurants are very, very big.

If you eat in restaurants a lot, cutting back on the portion sizes, eating fewer starchy carbs, and ordering dessert only for special occasions are essential patterns you need to start and turn into habits if you want to avoid or reverse Type 2 diabetes and lose weight.

Tips for Reducing Portion Size

By now you know the general guidelines for *what to eat*. So I'm going to focus on portion size, which I believe is the biggest problem for most of us when we eat dinner out.

Here are three effective ways to reduce portion size in restaurants:

1. Share the entrée with your dinner partner. This idea is becoming common especially with restaurant dinner customers in their 50s and older, but it's a good idea for anyone of any age who wants to lower blood sugars and lose weight. Some restaurants will, however, charge a second-plate fee but many do not.

2. Make an appetizer (or two) your dinner following the *Diabetes Lifeline* guidelines you now know. If you try this for a few months as a pattern and are able to let it evolve into a habit, you will have achieved a great health victory and be on your way to better blood sugar control, significant weight loss, and dramatically improved health. Make no mistake about this. It is hard. Your need to ask yourself how badly you want or need the positive results you will experience.

3. As you *place* your order, ask the server to put half the meal in a to-go container *before* he or *she brings it out to you*. You'll find it so much easier to eat only half of the overly generous plateful of food if you don't see the other half until you look in the refrigerator the next day.

A Final Thought on Seafood Restaurants and Butter

Seafood restaurants provide the best opportunity to illustrate a delicious way to enjoy good size servings of protein, vegetables, and fat with insignificant increases in blood sugar and weight.

As an example I'm going to use Red Lobster, a seafood restaurant that I eat at when I'm in California. Over the years I've eaten there I've confirmed—by consistent blood sugar testing before and after meals there—that I can eat all the lobster, prawns, scallops, salmon, halibut, and vegetables that I want with all the melted butter I want with almost negligible impact on my blood sugar and therefore on my weight.

However, once again, I must stress that all that changes if I eat starchy carbs with the meal or follow the meal with sweet carbs. But if you stay away from those two groups it's a wonderful way to enjoy a delicious, healthy meal.

Developing Active Habits

So far we've talked about what we put in our mouths. Now let's talk about how we can use the food more effectively before it gets stored.

Chapter 9

Walking— A Great Lifelong Activity

For Type 2 diabetics, pre-diabetics, borderline diabetics, or anyone who wants to lose weight and feel better

The Trick with Life is to Make it Look Easy.

—anonymous

Three lifestyle changes are important for anyone who wants to lower blood sugar, lose weight, and enjoy better health. The three lifestyle changes are as follows:

1. *Adopt a healthy eating lifestyle.* This is by far the most important of the three lifestyle changes based on my blood sugar tests.

2. *Embrace an active lifestyle.* This is the second most important of the three.

3. Embark on a simple, maintainable, healthy, *structured-exercise lifestyle.*

The previous chapters covered by far the most important of the three lifestyle changes necessary to lower blood sugar, lose weight and improve your health—*a healthy eating lifestyle.* This chapter covers the second most important lifestyle change—*an active lifestyle.*

Daily Activity

Based on blood sugar tests and resulting insulin demand, if I do well in the other two healthy lifestyles (eating and a structured exercise program) but am sedentary and don't walk the rest of the day, my insulin demand is about 20 percent higher which translates to a small incremental weight gain. I use the word "small" here because I'm referring to only one day. If you're a Type 2 diabetic trying to lower your blood sugar and lose weight without adding walking or other activity to your daily life, you can do that but it will be harder.

However, if you add activity and exercise lifestyle changes, you will improve your mobility, your posture, and your appearance. You'll not only have a longer life but you'll have a longer, healthy life.

This chapter is about stepping up the activity level in your daily life in ways you may never have thought of and making those new levels of activity your new active lifestyle. Daily activity is the easiest of the three lifestyle changes to make and the easiest to develop into habits. I'll teach you how to develop this new lifestyle while recognizing that many of you reading this book may have some significant limitations on what you can do now so we'll start slow and build from there.

Why So Many Other Nationalities are Slimmer Than Americans

Over the past 40 years, I've visited urban and rural areas in about 60 countries on six of the world's seven continents—I haven't been to Antarctica—and have come to realize that most of the world's people walk a lot more than Americans do. Some may say that we Americans are lazy. I disagree totally with that premise. How much people of different countries walk is due to factors far out of the control of most of the world's citizens—primarily the historical development and design of cities and the economic imperatives of countries—that determine whether people walk a lot or don't walk much.

Most European and Asian cities were far along in their development hundreds of years before automobiles replaced horses, oxen, and humans as the primary vehicles for moving goods and promoting commerce. The widths of the streets in Europe and Asia were designed to accommodate the needs of the time. Buildings were built hard on both sides of streets with little room for more than sidewalks and narrow streets for the relatively narrow, slow-moving carts. Adjusting for automobiles is now prohibitively expensive and destructive of cities' infrastructure. As a result, the narrow streets remain unaccommodating to automobile driving and parking. The result: people walk or ride bikes.

On Mary's and my first visit to China in 1980, our interpreters stated that Beijing had only 800 privately owned cars in the whole city of nine million people at that time. The result: millions of people walked or rode in a rolling sea of people and bicycles on every main street. Now Beijing has over 20 million people with hundreds of thousands of cars crawling in a perpetual traffic jam but because of the economic imperative of general poverty, millions of people still walk and ride their bikes.

In Paris, London, Prague, Lausanne and most other large European cities the sidewalks are bustling and flowing with walkers. Walking is necessary, of course, but also enjoyable for native citizens and visitors alike. Only Manhattan, in my experience in American cities, comes close to matching the walking requirements and experiences of European cities.

A few years ago, I spent a month in the African country of Malawi volunteering at an orphanage started by two longtime friends, Tom and Ruth Nighswander.

In Malawi, people walk for a different reason. Malawians have few cars and insufficient discretionary income to even dream of purchasing a car or fuel. Walking is the primary form of transportation and commerce. My mind's eye clearly recalls tall, slim, erect Malawian women walking in single lines with wooden branches, sacks of maize and jugs of water balanced firmly on top of their heads. This is the commerce of rural Malawi. This is their transportation system.

As you can guess, people in the areas I've just described are largely slim and healthy looking. Other factors may influence their apparent health but I believe walking is a significant contributor. The balance of this chapter will give you techniques to develop a pattern of walking more and making that pattern your lifelong habit.

Buy a Pedometer and Some Good "Around Home" Walking Shoes

I recommend that you buy what I call "around home walking shoes." Most of your walking is going to be around home, around the yard, around your neighborhood, shopping and doing errands, so buy shoes that you're comfortable wearing in those venues.

I also recommend buying a pedometer. Almost any sporting goods or outdoor store will have one and most are less than $20. You can also get more elaborate digital pedometers but you don't need that to get started.

The pedometer will measure with good accuracy how many steps you take in a day. For the most accurate results, you should attach it to a belt or the waist of your pants or skirt.

Once you get a pedometer it's important to keep a log of how many steps you're taking. Begin by establishing your baseline—how many steps you're taking now. It's best to do that for at least a week since some days, especially weekends, may vary from weekdays. Then use that baseline to compete with yourself. Each day try to beat the previous day's steps. After you've used it for a couple of weeks or so and have an idea of what you are doing and what you may be able to do in terms of steps per day, then you can start thinking about goals.

Here are some things to think about in your daily step's goal setting. Dr. Catrine Tudor-Locke published a study in 2004 involving 200 men and women. The men in the survey took an average of 7,192 steps a day and the women in the survey took an average of 5,210 steps.

In 2001, the U.S. Surgeon General, Dr. David Satcher issued "The Surgeon General's Call to Action to Prevent and Decrease Overweight and Obesity." The report recommended 30 minutes a day of moderate activity.

Most health experts seem to agree that 8,000–9,000 steps a day is an excellent healthy pattern to be in. That may sound daunting but I'm willing to bet that most of you will be surprised at how many steps you're already taking.

Whether your baseline is 1,000 steps a day, 3,000 steps, 5,000 steps or more, this suggestion is easy and very flexible. At the end of the first month you'll not only feel healthier but you'll also enjoy a feeling of physical pride that you may not have felt for a while.

Find a Friend to Walk with On a Regular Schedule

Finding a friend or friends to walk with is one of the best ways to build a regular walking habit. You'll have both company and commitment. You'll see things in your own neighborhood you never noticed from your car. You may end up stopping and talking to people who have lived near you for years but who you've never shared a story or even a greeting with. People who have enjoyed this habit for a long time talk about this time as a pleasant, satisfying part of their day.

Here are two stories of people in their 70s who have developed a habit of walking and maintained that habit for years—and all are healthy and trim.

My Sister, Rosanne, and Her Walking Friend, Dona Avila

Eighteen years ago my sister, Rosanne Bader, retired after a 32-year career as a teacher and principal in the Pomona Unified School District. Her friend, Dona Avila, an art teacher in the same district had retired a few years earlier. Once my sister retired, the two ladies committed to starting a walking program together.

The two women live just two houses away from each other at the top of a hilly area covered with nicely spaced homes fronted with cedar and foothill pines as well as oak, alder and cottonwoods. For nine months of the year flowering plants decorate their walks.

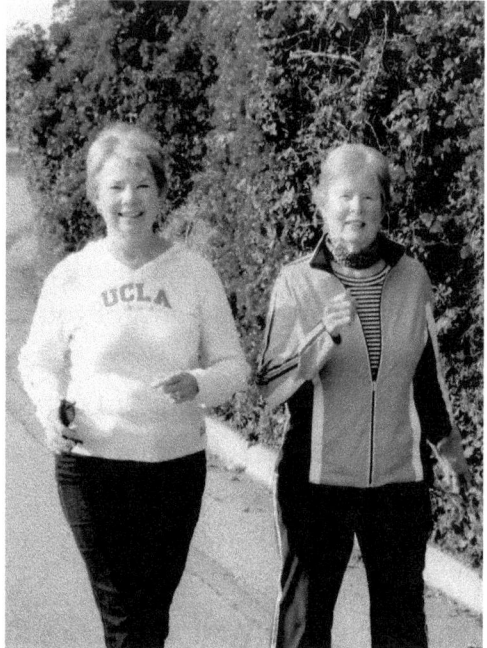

They made some early and lasting decisions about their walks that have served them well. They decided upon morning walks, "We start at 8 a.m." said Rosanne. We agreed to a Monday through Friday schedule and we simply call each other the night before if a morning meeting or commitment requires a cancellation of the day's walk," she added.

14 Year Walkers

Rosanne Bader on the left, and Dona Avila, have been walking the neighborhood hills in Pomona, California since they both retired from education careers 14 years ago.

Now, 18 years later, Rosanne talks warmly about their lifestyle habit. "Since our homes are at the top of the hill, we always start out downhill. We like to talk as we walk and at first we could only talk on the downhill half. Coming home uphill we just walked without talking—not because we didn't want to talk, we just couldn't walk uphill and talk at the same time. Now," she says, "we talk the whole way."

"It's just fun" she gushed. "We greet our neighbors, wave to the cars and pick up trash along the way. The 2.2 mile up and downhill walk seems to go by so fast."

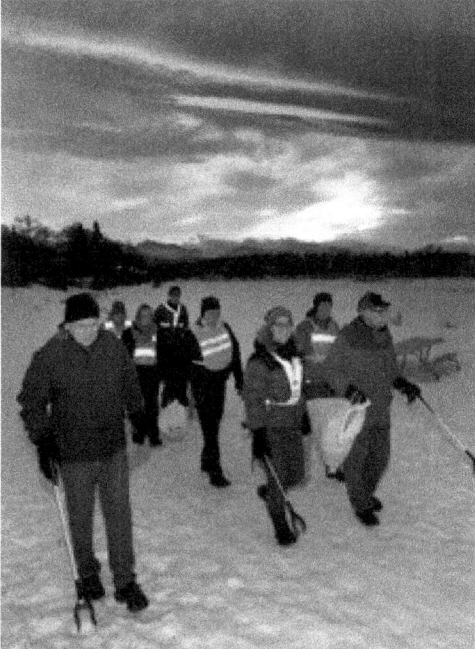

Five mornings a week—whether spring, summer, fall, or winter for about 38 years—this sociable and fit group of Anchorage citizens have been walking our neighborhoods and picking up trash.

It's no surprise that these "girls" are so trim and so healthy. Rosanne, by the way, is 76 and Dona is 83, and both look and feel great.

The Anchorage Trash Fairies

About nine years ago we moved to a new neighborhood, a few miles from where we had lived for over 35 years. Early in the morning as I was leaving for work or workout, I often saw a group of cheerful, physically fit neighbors walking, talking, laughing…and picking up litter. I knew some of them and asked how long they had been doing their early-morning excursions. Judy Sedwick, apparently one of the leaders, said, "Well, I started when my daughter was in kindergarten and now she's 43." They have a good active lifestyle, they're in excellent physical shape and our little part of the world is better because of them.

The Importance of After-Dinner Walking or Similar Activities

At no other time in your day will activity have as much impact on your blood sugar and weight as the hours between dinner and bedtime. This is the time our promises die. This is the time our health gets superseded by sloth unless we actively choose health. This is not just other people's problems. It was mine too for a few years and it may be yours now.

In the early 1990s, I was approaching 50 and I noticed a more sedentary after- dinner pattern showing up in my life during the winter months. The summer months were not a problem because of the long daylight hours in Alaska. I was almost always active and busy during those long sunny, summer evenings. More than once I recall my wife saying, "Rick, you'd better stop cutting the lawn; it's almost midnight and you'll disturb the neighbors."

For a couple of years, though, November through April was a different story. I found myself doing what I never thought I would do—surfing the television channels from about 9 p.m. to 11 p.m. It didn't take me long to realize I was not only wasting two hours of my life each night but I was also increasing my insulin requirement by about 20 percent. Remember increasing insulin demand means gaining weight.

After gaining weight and getting a little softer around my stomach, I decided to make two changes to my lifestyle. The first lifestyle change was to always shoot for at least 15 to 30 minutes of activity between dinner and bedtime. The second lifestyle change was to start going to bed earlier and begin waking up earlier. So instead of wasting two hours in nonproductive lethargy late at night I went to bed earlier, started waking up earlier and going to a health club for a light workout four or five days a week first thing in the morning.

Not only did the 15 to 30 minutes of activity reduce my insulin demand in the evening, but waking up early and working out started a long-term exercise pattern that continues in the winter months today.

Both of those changes had a very positive impact on my health, my physique, my insulin requirement, my blood sugar control, my weight, and my productivity.

I'll talk more about the importance of a moderate exercise program in the next chapter, but here I'll speak specifically about what you should do after dinner.

My Experiments with Insulin Reduction from After-Dinner Activity

When I first began to associate a rise in blood sugar and the resultant increased insulin demand with a lack of activity after dinner, I decided to try an experiment to prove or disprove the premise that a relatively small amount of activity after dinner and before bedtime can have a significant impact on blood sugar, insulin demand, and weight.

I decided the best way to establish the impact or lack of impact of activity after dinner was to eat the same or very similar dinners on consecutive nights and follow those dinners with either activity or inactivity before bedtime. I chose a dinner that I ate often and made a special point of trying to eat similar portion sizes.

It turned out my premise was valid. When I followed my similar meals with at least a half hour of some activity after dinner as simple as walking around the block, walking to a neighbor's home, or riding my bike around the neighborhood, I found that six or seven units of insulin was sufficient to balance that dinner. If I sat down in front of my computer or our TV set between dinner and bedtime and had virtually no activity, it would take nine to 10 units of insulin to balance that same meal. That's a significant reduction in insulin demand resulting from that modest activity between dinner and going to bed.

That reduced insulin demand meant less work for my pancreas and less weight gain—or weight loss—for the same meal.

That Small Amount of Activity Over a Year Translates into a Large Weight Loss

Let me explain the impact of that activity in another way. The roughly two to three units of additional insulin I needed to take when I had no activity after dinner is about the same amount of insulin I would take to balance a standard size Hershey bar, which is a little more than 200 calories. Not having any activity after dinner was like adding the equivalent of a candy bar to my dinner.

Having no activity after dinner every day for a year is like adding 365 candy bars to your calorie intake. If you assume a candy bar is about 200 calories, that's roughly a 75,000-calorie impact over a year. Every pound of fat is equivalent to about 3,500 calories, which means those 75,000 calories added—because of inactivity—over 20 pounds of fat per year.

Continuation of Fat Burning When You're Asleep

Now conventional wisdom would say that 30 minutes of light to moderate activity is insufficient to burn 200 calories, but conventional wisdom hasn't been tested like this. My observation is that a continuation effect of calorie burning takes effect and a slight increase in metabolism continues prior to bedtime and for the first hour or more of your sleep.

My conclusion based on the specifics of insulin demand is that some activity between the time you eat and the time you go to bed is the *most important and effective activity you will have all day.*

The first thing you need to do is to get into the mindset of moving after dinner. If you're one of those folks who gets up from the table, moves to the living room and positions yourself in front of a TV or a computer, changing that pattern and adding about a half hour of some physical movement after dinner will have a big impact on your weight and health.

So how do you get into the habit of doing this?

After-Dinner Activity Suggestions

1. Do some of your daily "out of home" chores after dinner instead of doing them before dinner. For example, do your food shopping and any other shopping or errands after dinner and when you do it, park farther away from the store than you normally do.

2. Instead of doing yard work on weekends, do a little bit each evening after dinner.

3. Get in a habit of taking an after-dinner walk with friends or your spouse. It doesn't have to be long. It can be just around the block to start and let it build naturally to longer walks. This is different from a morning walk. It doesn't have to be as long to be effective in reducing the glucose created by your dinner.

4. If you go out to eat in a location that accommodates walking, get in the habit of parking three or four blocks away from the restaurant and walking to the restaurant. That action means you'll walk before you eat and more importantly after you eat.

5. If you have a shopping mall nearby, go there and walk around for a while.

6. When you do sit down in front of the TV, make it a point to get up and walk around your house or yard during commercials. This will also help you curtail snacking because a commercial break is one of the most common snacking cues.

Conclusion
You don't have to work hard after dinner, just move. You're going to move naturally after breakfast and lunch but you don't necessarily move after dinner. You should begin this pattern and make it your habit. You will be astounded at the difference this will make in your weight and health over the years.

This Is Not an Activity but It Works—
Lower the Temperature in Your Bedroom
at Night by a Couple of Degrees
At first I was perplexed by some differences I noted in my morning blood sugars because I'm a believer that all blood sugar levels have reasons behind them. I couldn't figure out why, when I went to bed with my blood sugar stable –no insulin or food going in—at 110 or 120 , I sometimes woke up with a blood sugar very close to that and sometimes with a blood sugar 50 or 60 points lower. It took me 20 years to recognize that the drop of 50 or 60 points in my blood sugar was related to the temperature in the room I was sleeping in. The lower the temperature the more glucose my body burned trying to keep warm and the more my blood sugar dropped.

You mean I'm going to lose weight while I'm sleeping? The answer is yes you will. This is not really an activity but it's an action. Think about it this way. Let's say you like your indoor temperature at 70 degrees. If you heat your house with natural gas and say the temperature is 50 degrees outside, you'll be burning some amount of gas to make up that 20-degree difference to keep your house at 70 degrees. If the next night, the temperature goes down to 40 degrees, are you going to use more gas than the night before to keep your house at 70 degrees because you've got a 30-degree difference to make up instead of 20 degrees? Yes. You will burn more gas to make up that 30-degree difference.

Your body's like a house—well, actually, I hope not. It works hard to keep its temperature at 98.6 degrees Fahrenheit. The greater the difference (lower only) between the ambient temperature outside your body and 98.6 degrees, the more glucose your body must burn to heat itself. For example, if you keep your bedroom temperature at 70 degrees, that's a difference of 28.6 degrees your body need to make up. If you lower your bedroom temperature at night to 68 degrees, the difference your body will have to make up is 30.6 degrees.

Now you may put on more blankets to keep warmer—try not to do that— but your face (and in my case my head) will still be exposed. Some extra calories will be burned.

Now 50 points on my blood sugar doesn't exactly relate to 50 calories but coincidentally it's close. To give you an idea about what that means in terms of food—for me this is about the amount of weight I'd gain by eating a third of a typical candy bar or by drinking a quarter of a can of sugared soda every day. I know that because that's what I would have to eat or drink to raise my blood sugar about 50 points.

How Much Difference Can Lowering Bedroom Temperature Make in a Person's Weight in a Year?

Think about this from another angle. If two people my size (6'3", 190 lbs) lived in adjoining apartments and one kept the bedroom at 68 degrees, the other at 70 degrees, the one in the warmer bedroom pays a weight gain penalty each night of the equivalent of eating a third of a candy bar each day.

You may say "a third of a candy bar"? That's no big deal". But think about the impact it would have over time. A third of a candy bar a day is roughly two candy bars a week or 100 candy bars a year. Now you've got to believe 100 candy bars a year will make a difference in your weight.

Using the calculations earlier in this chapter about the impact of activity after dinner, subtracting about 100 candy bars from your annual intake subtracts about 20,000 calories or about the equivalent of about six pounds per year. That habit over a 10-year period is in the ball park of 60 pounds saved.

This action falls into the category of pretty easy to do and will have a small short-term impact but a meaningful, cumulative impact over the years. However, if lowering your bedroom temperature negatively impacts your sound sleep, don't do it. A good night's sleep is priceless and this book contains lots of other lifestyle options that will result in weight loss and better health.

Chapter 10

A Moderate and Sustainable Strength-Building Program

The Type 2 Workout Program

The Importance of a Moderate Exercise Lifestyle

This chapter covers the last of the three lifestyle changes you need embrace to lower your blood sugars, lose weight, and live a longer, healthier life. By way of review, developing a *healthy eating lifestyle* is the most important lifestyle change you can make. Creating an *active lifestyle* and adopting a *structured exercise lifestyle* are the final two lifestyle changes needed to live a long, healthy life.

Your goal should be to start this as a program, make it a pattern, let it evolve into a habit and then make it a continuing part of your lifestyle.

This program, "The Type 2 Exercise Program" is designed for Type 2 diabetics who may never have taken part in a structured exercise program or who may not have exercised for a long time. It's a simple, short program that starts out very slowly and non-strenuously and allows you to match your workout to your strength—or lack of strength—and increase the weights as strength and fitness allow. As you will see, the key element in this program is never to work so hard that you don't want to do it the next day. I want you to feel good—not feel worn out—after you complete each workout.

Although this program is designed primarily for Type 2 diabetics, it will also be very helpful for anyone, overweight or not, who would like to have a simple, structured, sustainable exercise program as part of his or her life.

The beauty of adding this program to your lifestyle is the addition of aerobic health *and* muscular gain.

The aerobic health you'll achieve will be beneficial to your heart and circulatory system and includes myriad other benefits you can read about in any of the hundreds of books about aerobic sports.

The strength-gain element of the exercise program I'm recommending also has multiple benefits. To start with, whether you're a man or a woman, having a higher ratio of muscle to fat in your body means you'll burn more calories in your daily life than a person of the same sex and size who has less muscle than you do. This means that you can eat the same amount and types of food as this other person and gain less weight or lose more weight than he or she will. Other benefits include increased strength, better posture, better mobility for longer, and less fragility as you age. And—by the way—you'll look better. You will experience these benefits by making the strength training element a part of your exercise lifestyle.

Remember that exercise and activity work like insulin to lower the blood sugar. That means your blood sugar will go down and relieve your overworked pancreas of having to produce so much insulin.

When you combine all three of these elements—*eating the right food, embracing a more active lifestyle, and starting a moderate exercise program,* you will lower your blood sugars, eliminate all symptoms of diabetes, and likely eliminate all need for diabetes medications.

Why This Exercise Program Is Different from All the Others

How many times in your life have you heard the terms, "Give it your all," "No pain, no gain," "Go the extra mile," or "Don't quit now." If you haven't competed in a lot of sports, you may not have heard these motivational missives at all but believe me, they're very common in America and probably many other countries. I see people (mostly guys) every week in gyms living these guidelines. They're lifting heavy weights. They're grunting. They're yelling. They're sweating and … they usually disappear within a few weeks. Not always though. If they're training for a competition, they may be doing the right thing and they may very well persist until the competition. But if they expect it to be a lifetime health and fitness habit, it won't work.

Who *This Type 2 Exercise Program Is Not* For

Walk past any supermarket magazine rack and you'll see dozens of fitness magazines for men and women. Probably 90 percent of the photos focus on abs (stomach muscles) and all of them have pictures of men and women with beautifully toned and hard lean muscles with little body fat. Many of the serious muscle magazines show bizarre-looking, overly muscled behemoths. If your goal is to look like these men and women, **this program is not for you**. To look like these magazine cover photos, here's what you would have to do. Pay attention to what I said about food and then add about 200 grams of additional protein to your daily diet. Then find a good trainer and commit to spending about 10 to 20 hours a week in strength and aerobic training. When you've done all that find a photographer who's good at photoshop and can take away the blemishes and any remaining fat.

Who This Program *Is* For

However, if your goal is to lower your blood sugar, lose weight, lower your blood pressure, feel better, and look better, **this program *is* for**

you. Beyond your body looking better, your face will look better as you lose fat. As we gain weight, our faces become rounder and lose the definition we had when we were thinner. As we lose weight the definition slowly and subtly begins the return trip to our faces.

If you're a woman, in addition to the above, you can expect to reduce your dress size, pant size, improve your posture, and cut inches off your hips and legs.

If you're a guy—I've learned I can call a man a guy but calling a woman a gal, the parallel equivalent, is offensive to some—in addition to the above, you can expect to increase the size of your shoulders, arms, and chest, decrease the size of your stomach and improve your posture.

Because this program is not an intense program, it will work for any Type 2 diabetic from an overweight preteen to an optimistic 85-year-old great-grandpa who still wants to chase women even if it's only downhill, or to the 90-year-old "girl" who still wants to look and feel better.

This is my program. I've used it for the past 15 years and it's worked beautifully. It's simple, clear, easy to start and easy to maintain. Adding this simple exercise program to the first two elements—a healthy eating lifestyle and an active lifestyle--will result in a complete fitness lifestyle. Starting these lifestyles is the beginning. Lifetime fitness is the ending.

The Basics of the Type 2 Diabetics' Workout Program

This Type 2 workout program is designed for people who have not exercised on a regular basis for years or maybe have never exercised. It's a simple program to get you into a gym and keep you coming back. If you don't belong to a gym or health club or have one nearby, you can still follow the patterns I'm proposing by purchasing some basic equipment or if you choose, more elaborate equipment, to use at home.

Here's the basic philosophy of the Type 2 Diabetics' Exercise Program:

1. The program requires and rewards persistence, not intensity. It may be as little as 20 minutes three days a week or as much as 40 minutes six days a week—or somewhere in between.

2. You'll include strength training and aerobics in your daily workout starting at a level appropriate to your existing condition and ability.

3. You'll start slowly and never work so hard on any given day that you don't want to do it again the next day.

4. You'll start every series of repetitions (reps) with weights light enough to allow you to repeat a motion 35 times (35 reps). I'll explain why later in this chapter.

5. You'll never use a weight so heavy that you can't do 15 reps.

6. You should approach this as a one-year program. By the end of that time you'll be a fitter, healthier person and you'll know what works for you so you can determine your own future program adjustments.

7. As you begin this program, you should increase protein consumption to give your muscles the fuel to grow. Protein has little impact on your blood sugar but a lot of impact on muscle growth and fitness.

8. If you can maintain this program for three months, you will be well on your way to making it part of your everyday life and a final step in your new healthy lifetime lifestyle.

Getting Started with your Aerobic Workout

Your aerobic workout is very simple. Most gyms have three or four options and if a gym doesn't work for you, walking or riding a bike can achieve the same goals.

In a gym, your workout can take place on a stationary bike, a treadmill, a stair climber, or an elliptical trainer. Do only what you're comfortable with. You may be able to start by walking on a treadmill or riding a stationary bike for only 10 minutes; that's fine. Remember not to push yourself. This is the beginning of a long, pleasant journey and if you work too hard at first you'll likely make it only a short journey.

If you're using a machine that measures calories you burn start with a 10-minute workout and see how many calories you burn. During your first week stay with that number of calories. Each week increase the calories by an amount you can manage. You can also increase the time but don't go beyond 20 minutes. Combining 20 minutes of aerobics with 20 minutes of strength training nears the threshold for most people beyond which making it a daily habit becomes difficult. The best is to stay at 10 minutes aerobic and 20 minutes of strength training. If you're doing a lot of walking outside the gym, then just use the gym only for strength training.

Remember a key to an effective exercise lifestyle is to never work so hard—or so long—that you don't want to come back the next day.

Getting Started with Your Strength Workout

Many of you may never have done any strength workouts so we'll start with the very basics. Most strength workout programs deal with very specific muscles and muscle groups, with muscle terms like "delts" (deltoid muscles), "lats" (latissimus dorsi), "pecs" (pectoralis), "traps" (trapezius), "abs" (abdominal muscles) and many more muscles and muscle groups. The Type 2 Fitness Program simplifies all this by dividing your strength workout into three categories.

The Type 2 Diabetes Lifeline Program Deals with Only Three Categories

The three categories you'll work are very simply *your front, your core, and your back*. Using these categories dramatically simplifies the daily workout but still covers all the parts of your body needed for muscle enhancement, improvement in the ratio of muscle to fat, and posture and appearance improvement.

This is the program I've used for the past 15 years and it has served me very well. I have not done specific leg exercises but rather have counted on my eating and activity lifestyle to keep my legs in shape. More women than men seem to focus on adding strength workouts for their legs and that's simply a personal choice you can make. Although women tend to gain weight on their legs and hips more commonly than men do, healthy eating combined with more activity will promote losing inches on hips and legs. Men are more prone to gain their weight on their bellies and often adapt to this problem by simply moving the front of their pants down inch by inch, year by year.

For both men and women exercising "abs" will make those muscles stronger but it will not make your stomach slimmer, or your waist smaller, or your abs more defined. What will make your stomach slimmer and your waist smaller, and your abs more defined is combining your new healthy eating and activity lifestyles with your "abs" exercises.

The Importance of Eating More Protein

Before I outline the workout program, I'm going to talk once again about food—in this case protein. About 15 years ago when I first began my workout program with my fitness trainer, Philip Bradfield, I noticed two other men working out as partners every morning at the same time. They appeared to be in their late 40s or early 50s. One was quite muscular with not much body fat. He was the workout leader of the two. The other man, the follower, was much less muscular with an average-looking body and a moderate amount of body fat.

When Philip and I were in the gym for our sessions, I noted that these guys never talked to each other. They walked with purpose—sometimes bordering on what seemed like anger—from one machine to another. They alternated attacks on the machines. Grunting, pushing, yelling, and sweating. Generally working four or five times harder than I did during the time I was there. Every morning they were there driving themselves and each other with a passion that seemed to me to be impossible to sustain.

After a couple of months, they were—surprisingly—still at it. I pulled Philip aside and said, "As hard as these guys are working, I haven't seen a bit of change in the 'follower,' the guy with the average build."

It was true. That guy had been killing himself for months and nothing changed.

Philip responded. "He's not eating right. His body has nothing to build with—no protein." He went on. "Usually people who work that hard and don't see results because they're not eating right, quit within the first month. He's lasted longer than most but he'll get discouraged and quit pretty soon when he realizes nothing's happening."

The message is this: If you want to see and feel results from your workouts, you need to increase the amount of protein you eat. Try to eat more eggs or egg whites (either is fine), more fish, and other seafood, more chicken, pork, beef, steak or hamburger. Some vegetables are also high in protein. As you develop your exercise program, you'll have more noticeable results if you eat more of these high-protein vegetables: spinach, peas, broccoli, and artichokes.

Remember protein has very little impact on your blood sugar and the vegetables I mentioned, even though they do have some carbohydrates, also have very little impact on your blood sugar. Eat more of these proteins and fewer starchy carbs and sweet carbs and you will gain muscle and lose fat from workouts.

The Importance of "Front," "Core," and "Back" Workouts

Day one—Work on the **front** part of your body (anterior shoulders, chest and biceps). This muscle grouping is important for strength, appearance, and increasing muscle-to-fat ratio.

Day two—Work on the **core** part of your body (abdominal muscles, lower back muscles, and side muscles). This muscle grouping is very important in tying the upper part of your body to the lower part. They add athleticism and grace to your movement and aid significantly in avoiding back problems for men and women. Men tend to have more back problems than women because with generally more upper body strength we tend to try and lift heavier objects. We're also generally a little taller which puts more force on a lifting motion than a shorter person experiences. Back problems can be diminished or avoided by strengthening core muscles.

Day three—Work on the **back** part of your body (upper back, triceps, and midback). This muscle grouping is usually the most ignored in many people's exercise programs. They are however, very important for balance, erectness, and back health. Working only on the front muscles and ignoring the back results in a rolled-forward, slouching posture that is unhealthy and unattractive. Back workouts are a friend of good posture and good appearance.

Focusing each day on different parts of your body as I've described has three distinct advantages:

First, for those people who have not done any strength training this is very easy to categorize and remember where you are on any given day. For example, "today is my day for front or for core or for 'back." You don't have to work so hard to recall the muscles worked on over the past few days.

Second, your muscles will get an automatic two-day rest between the times they are worked. Having at least one or two days for muscle rest and growth is the one thing almost all strength-training gurus agree on. This program gives your muscles a two-day rest.

Third, the program works simply and beautifully with a three-day or six-day workout plan. I've found that it's easier to maintain this program if you take at least one day a week off.

The Patterns to Follow on All Three Days

Start Very Light

Start with a weight resistance that will allow you to do 35 repetitions. This will probably be a very light weight. For some it may be as light as five pounds for others it may be 40 or more pounds.

This high number of repetitions is very important for people who have not exercised for a long time. You'll see I focus on the number of times (repetitions) you should do and not the weight you should use. By focusing on repetitions, you will automatically choose the appropriate weight for your level of strength.

The reason for the high number of repetitions is to allow your muscle to warm up. This warming up does two things.

First, it prevents injuries like adhesive tendinitis, an irritation of the tendons which attach bone to muscle. If you don't start with very light resistance, you will feel tiny, almost imperceptible pops in the muscles you are working. These are little threads of tendons tearing.

These micro tears won't hurt but they do cause a release of fluid that when it dries acts like super glue. Enough of these small tears will begin to restrict your range of motion to the extent that it will prevent your ability to reach behind your back or neck, so even putting on a shirt, blouse, or jacket can hurt.

Second, by warming up sufficiently you will be able to do subsequent repetitions with heavier weights and therefore better results.

Increase Your Weights for the Next Two Sets

Next, move to heavier weights or resistance that allows you to do 25 repetitions. This is still a high number of repetitions so it should not be enough resistance to tear any tendons.

Finally, increase the weight or resistance to a level that will allow you to do 15 repetitions.

The weight or resistance you choose will be determined by the number of repetitions you are able to do. Your sets of 15 reps will be with a heavier weight than your sets of 25 and your sets of 25 will be with heavier than your sets of 35. You'll never need to increase those numbers of repetitions but you will find with great satisfaction that within the first month you will naturally begin using heavier weights and more resistance for the same number of repetitions.

The Type 2 Workout Calendar

DAY ONE

You may opt to start with a 10-minute light aerobic workout described above followed by a "front" strength workout below.

Front (Anterior Muscles)

AUTHOR'S NOTE:

Biceps

35 Repetitions with a starting weight of your choice

25 Reps with a slightly heavier weight

15 Reps with a heavier weight

Remember the weights are determined by your ability to do the number of Reps called for. You may increase by increments as small as five pounds or as much as 20 or 30 pounds.

Chest

35 Reps with a starting weight of your choice

25 Reps with a slightly heavier weight

15 Reps with a heavier weight

Anterior Shoulders

35 Reps with a starting weight of your choice

25 Reps with a slightly heavier weight

15 Reps with a heavier weight

You're done with your Day One strength workout.

DAY TWO

Again you may opt to start with your aerobic workout followed by the "core" strength workout below.

Core

Abdominal Muscles (Abs)

(The same pattern as day one)

35 Reps with a starting weight or resistance of your choice

25 Reps with a slightly heavier weight

15 Reps with a heavier weight

Lower Back

35 Reps with starting weight or resistance of your choice

25 Reps with a slightly heavier weight

15 Reps with increased weight

Side Muscles

35 Reps with a starting weight or resistance of your choice

25 Reps with a slightly heavier weight

15 Reps with a heavier weight

You're now done with your Day Two strength workout.

DAY THREE

Optional aerobic workout followed by the "back" workout below.

Back (Posterior Muscles)

Triceps

35 Reps with a starting weight or resistance of your choice
25 Reps with a slightly heavier weight
15 Reps with a heavier weight

Upper Back and Shoulders

35 Reps with a starting weight or resistance of your choice
25 Reps with a slightly heavier weight
15 Reps with a heavier weight

Mid-Back

35 Reps with a starting weight or resistance of your choice
25 Reps with a slightly heavier weight
15 Reps with a heavier weight

You're now done with your three-day strength workout.

Choose a Six-day-per-Week or Three-day-per-Week Schedule

If you choose to work out six days a week, repeat this pattern for days four, five, and six. Each muscle grouping will get two workouts in a week and two days of muscle rest before that group is worked again. Take the seventh day off and resume the pattern the following week.

If you choose to work out three days a week, simply repeat this pattern every other day with the seventh day off.

You'll find this is a simple pattern can become a habit and then a lifestyle. When you combine this exercise lifestyle with your new healthy eating lifestyle and more active lifestyle, you will lose weight, be healthier, feel stronger, look better and generally enjoy your life more.

Getting Started

The descriptions of the machines to use and an explanation of the techniques for using them do not lend themselves well to a book like this one. The best thing to do is to go to a health club and ask for direction on using the machines. The danger there is that some young trainer may try to talk you into working harder and lifting heavier. Don't do it. Follow the pattern I've described.

Another option is to go online or pick up a book with photos of working different muscle groups. Just be sure to ignore all the advice about how hard you should work and how heavy you should lift.

Comments on Past Presentations

By Rick Mystrom

Rick Mystrom has spoken nationwide at diabetes events, hospital seminars, annual meetings of businesses, Rotary clubs and many other service clubs.

You may contact him at:

> WEBSITE: Rick Mystrom.com
> EMAIL: mystrom@gci.net
> PHONE: 907-440-7425

"Rick Mystrom was a terrific speaker.
He had great clarity in his presentation.
It was personal, practical, and enjoyable."

"Number seven speaker, (Mystrom), was wonderful."

"I Enjoyed Rick Mystrom. He was very encouraging and upbeat."

"Please repeat Rick Mystrom's—*What Should I Eat* presentation. We missed it and were told it was excellent."

"Really liked the mayor from Alaska, Rick Mystrom"

"Rick Mystrom was the best." "Excellent." "Awesome"

"I like surprises. Rick Mystrom's, *What Should I Eat,* presentation was a delightful surprise."

"When you have speakers like Rick, who have so much to share, please allow them more time."

"I've been a nurse for 32 years. This was the best presentation on healthy eating I've ever seen."

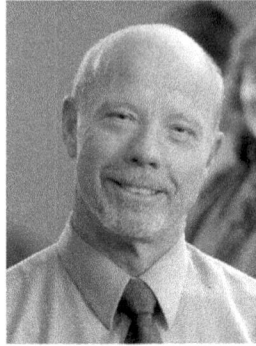

About the Author

Rick is a paragon of good health and has had Type 1 diabetes for 53 years. A recent stress test categorized him as equivalent to an "active 42-year-old." He credits his good health to good eating habits, an active lifestyle, and an understanding of foods. For over 35 years, he has tested his blood 5 to 10 times a day and has a unique understanding of which foods contribute to good health and which detract from good health.

For the past three years, Rick has meticulously measured, organized and graphed—in a way never before done—the impact that different foods and combination of foods have on blood sugar and weight gain or loss.

That information in this book means lower blood sugar and weight loss for Type 2 diabetics and better blood sugar control for Type 1 diabetics. And for the two thirds of all American adults who are anywhere between slightly overweight and obese, this book is your answer to a longer, healthier, more enjoyable life.

www.ingramcontent.com/pod-product-compliance
Lightning Source LLC
Chambersburg PA
CBHW071651200326
41519CB00012BA/2473